Medicine Reflections

Acknowledgement

This book was made possible by the support of a SEED Fund "Innovation in Teaching" grant (2017), from the Centre for Learning and Research in Higher Education at The University of Auckland. It was awarded to T. Jowsey, J. Yielder, S. Esteves, and R. Yielder; for which we are very grateful.

Jowsey, T. (Ed.) 2017. Medicine Reflections. Compassion Publishers: Auckland, New Zealand. Copyright 2017.

ISBN-13: 978-0-9874920-5-0

Cover image detail

Front cover: Coll Campbell, Year 4, *Tui Forest Lore*, 2016.
Back cover: James Corbett, Year 4, *Coming Together of Clinical Medicine*, 2016.

Contents

Biographical notes on key contributors

Dr Glenn Colquhoun is a poet and General Practitioner (GP). He works at a youth health service in Horowhenua, New Zealand.

Dr Sharyn Esteves qualified as a doctor 25 years ago and currently works as a Palliative Care doctor. Sharyn co-ordinates the Personal and Professional Skills Domain within the MBChB programme at The University of Auckland. Outside of work she has many creative interests that include painting, etching, mixed media and textiles.

Dr Tanisha Jowsey, PhD, is a medical anthropologist, lecturer, artist and writer at The University of Auckland. Tanisha has exhibited her works in art galleries in Australia and New Zealand, in four group and seven solo exhibitions (2001-2011). Some of her written works include *Musings from an Academic Kiwi* (Compassion Publishers 2016), *Chronic illness: the temporal thief* (Lambert 2016), and *Turtles and Diggers* (Compassion Publishers 2016).

Dr Art Nahill is a General Physician (Internal Medicine Physician) at Auckland City Hospital and a lover of poetry, committed to the idea that medicine and the arts are complementary parts of the same whole.

Associate Professor Ping Qu is a lecturer at Harbin Medical University, China. Ping has a long-term interest in developing students' empathy and critical reflective writing through narrative medicine.

Associate Professor Lisa Samuels is a transnational poet and essayist whose recent books are *Tender Girl* (2015), *Over Hear: six types of poetry experiment in Aotearoa/New Zealand* (2015), and *A TransPacific Poetics* (2017, edited with Sawako Nakayasu). Born in Boston, Lisa has lived since 2006 in Tāmaki Makaurau/Auckland. She teaches literature, theory, and creative writing at The University of Auckland.

Dr Jill Yielder, PhD, is Co-ordinator and teacher in the Personal & Professional Skills domain of the MBChB programme at The University of Auckland. Jill is also a Jungian Analyst and psychotherapist in private clinical practice. Her research interests include projects that support the PPS domain, other curriculum innovations and personality type/learning styles.

Ms Rachael Yielder, BA (Majoring in Psychology and Sociology), is currently studying Music Business in Manchester, UK. Rachael has a strong interest in all aspects of art and artist development.

Prologue

Glenn Colquhoun

What should I say? I have been asked to write a prologue to this collection and so I have read it and it makes me want to smile. It makes me recognise my own desire to write as a young man. It makes me want to say well done. And thank you. To those of you who have contributed, there you are, bright and shining, part of a tradition that stretches all the way back to Hippocrates and St Luke through to Keats and Chekhov and Williams Carlos Williams. You practice medicine and you write. I read some stuff about how to do this. It was wise and you should listen to it. But I want to say above everything else to keep doing what you are doing. Reach out. Watch. Listen. Feel. Be. Poems sweep out of the fury no doubt. But so often they rise with the cleaners when everyone else has left the room. Go back and sit with them. Take the words that float. Be strict. Don't hurry. Wait.

Sometimes we write to discover what we think. Poems are about words for sure, and craft. But there is something more to them than that. And medicine is about making people better. But there is something more to it than that as well. There are connections between people that are not readily seen. We pass beside each other so quickly. But in medicine there are wounds. Someone has stopped by the side of the road. Landscapes open in them that they do not always understand. Somewhere in these mists there are pathways. They zig-zag and are swept away in places, the width of man. They disappear in the mountains. They cross rivers. They stretch out across the plains. Find them and you will not only find another. You will find your own living staring back. You will find all of our living. Sometimes it is enough to acknowledge this and wonder. Patients want us to do this. Even if they do not know it. When we do a great and powerful tenderness is able to pass between us. That tenderness is not the everyday tenderness of making beds and taking blood pressures. It is something older. It is the recognition that we are tied together.

This is another sort of medicine altogether. It gives no guarantee that anyone will be cured or live forever. That is not its business. Not at all. Poems are found at this intersection too. They bring us to it, this edge between things where our skin dissolves. That is why they are useful. They teach us to be. This is the heart of writing. It is the heart of medicine too. Not words. Not needles.

I found something of this in your writing. Sometimes it was sitting on the end of a sentence or poking out sideways. Sometimes it was there despite the writing, separate from the craft. It made me smile. Keep going. Make room for it. Don't let it be buried. It will stand you in good stead. In medicine. And in writing. Thank you for your tenderness and for thinking to look at what each of you has looked at. This is more a mihi than a prologue.

You are my brothers and sisters twice over. Come for a cuppa sometime. I wish you such good things in this remarkable world.

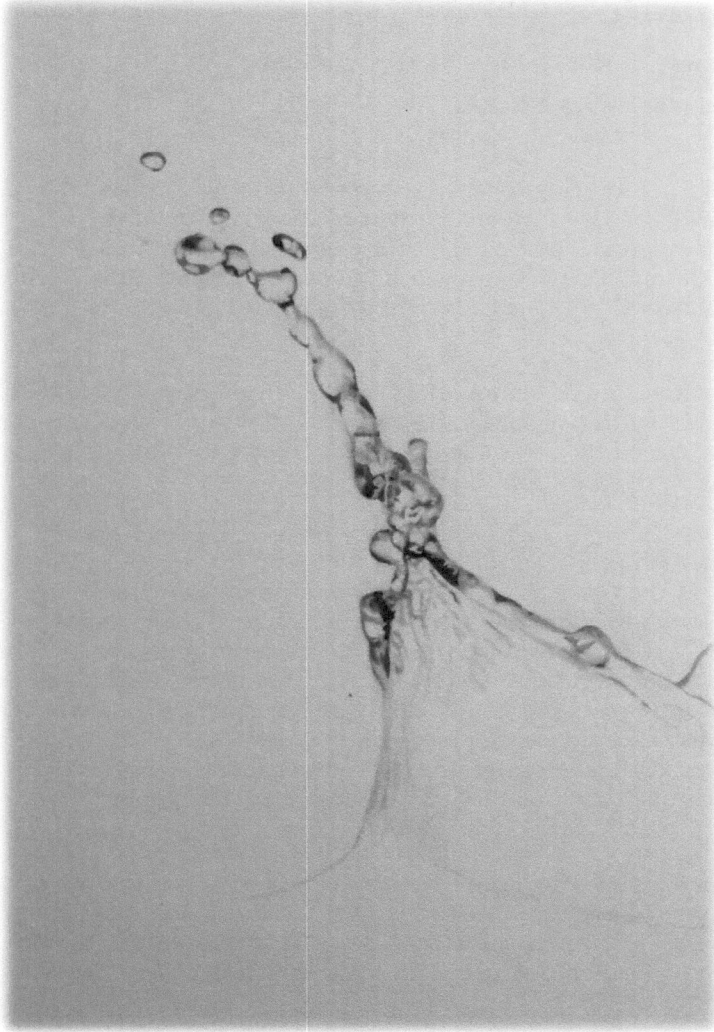

Chloe Bangs, Year 4, *Water Splash*, sketch on paper.

Introduction

Tanisha Jowsey, Jill Yielder, Sharyn Esteves,

Rachael Yielder and Art Nahill

We are delighted to bring to you this collection of 89 poems and 13 art works from 64 students undertaking a medical degree at the University of Auckland. Students from Years 4 and 5 of our programme in 2016 created these works to form our inaugural publication, and we hope it will be the first of many wonderfully reflective and insightful collections.

We have created this collection of works with the hopes that it will inspire students and health care practitioners, and that it will offer future students examples of the kinds of spaces into which they can take their own critical reflection and creative explorations.

As part of the Personal & Professional Skills (PPS) domain in the medical curriculum at the University of Auckland, students prepare reflective Portfolios. They are required to prepare evidence of their critical reflection for each of the five themes included in the domain (professionalism and reflective practice, ethics and the law, health and well-being, cultural competence, and teaching and learning). One element upon which the Portfolios are assessed is *creativity and engagement*. Students have demonstrated high levels of creativity and engagement in their portfolios through various mediums, often through poetry and art.

Narrative medicine is a genre of creative reflective writing that concerns itself with health-related experiences. Writing formats typically associated with narrative medicine include poetry, medical fiction, the lay exposition, autobiography, and stories from (clinical) practice.

While it can take various forms, such as those listed above, at its core is **an intention to facilitate critical reflection on clinical practice and to develop empathy**; between the clinical practitioner and their patients, and between the practitioner-writer and the reader. Other commonly-explored areas within narrative medicine include morals, ethics, difficult lived experiences, and tensions between systems and personal beliefs and practices.

These explored spaces are critical to shaping people's clinical practices of care and have been included in The University of Auckland Medical Programme, assessed by the Portfolio; "[t]he domain and the portfolio were introduced to Years 2 and 4 of the [medical] program in 2013, Years 3 and 5 in 2014, and Year 6 in 2015." (1) Now well underway, the PPS domain and Portfolios provide "an opportunity and incentive for students to reflect on aspects of their **personal and professional development**, with the aim of improving their practice as doctors."(1) It is thus intertwined with professionalism.

There is good evidence that the Portfolios offer students opportunities to increase their ability to critically reflect on, and engage with important elements of clinical practice. The outcomes are important for them in terms of their practice of patient-centred care and ongoing development of professionalism. Although there is no standard definition of medical professionalism, there is a consensus that it "signifies a set of values, behaviours and relationships that underpins the trust the public has in doctors" (Royal College of Physicians 2005), with attributes including compassion and **empathy**, resilience, advocacy, self-care and self-awareness. Within medical curricula globally, there is an increasing focus on the teaching and assessment of professionalism, although no consensus on how this is best done. Increasingly, students are being asked to creatively engage in reflective practice through the completion of Portfolios and other humanities teaching.

The five themes of learning included in the PPS domain

Professionalism and Reflective Practice

Ethics and the Law

Cultural Competence

Health and Well-being

Learning and Teaching.

University of Auckland Medical Programme: PPS Domain

Our students have focused largely on poetry and stories from clinical practice in their narrative medicine contributions to their Portfolios. Poetry is an excellent medium through which people can present their critical reflections on their experiences and imaginings. It invites creativity, and its many formats offer the poet a vast suite of options to choose from in terms of structure; from prose to ballads to sonnets, and everything in between.

The art submitted in the Portfolios typically includes photographs, paintings, illustrations or mindfulness colouring. These images are often included to illustrate how students balance their academic, clinical and home lives, how they relieve stress, or as a way of making sense of personal or clinical moments. The 13 original art works included here provide a visual aspect to frame this poetry collection.

So many artistic enquiries begin – and possibly end – with subjective sense-making of the world around us. We create art as part of – and in response to – this sense-making. We tell stories in an intersubjective dialectic.(2) We draw our visions. We move, dance, make noise, make food, and respond in creative diversity. Our very experience of existence flavours these artistic enterprises.

And so it is that in creating and responding to art, we often begin with existential ponderings. Who am I? What do I think? What do I feel? What is my experience? To what extent is my experience similar to those of others? How can my experience be portrayed, explored, conveyed visually? Or, how does this person's art speak to me? How can I make sense of this art?

Philosophy and art are thus intertwined.

Add to this time, space, and sociocultural facets, and we have yet more complexity. Can cave drawings in France that are thousands of years old speak to us in relevant ways today? Are cubism and post-modern art constructs that should inform our sense-making?

Is art "anything you can get away with"?(3)

Or is it, as Kamhi suggests, **"visual imagery that skilfully represents real or imagined people, places, and things in a form expressive of the maker's temperament, deeply held values, and view of life"?**(3)

Our students, whose art works are presented in this collection, have grappled with philosophy, subjectivity and artistic discourse through their art works. They have used visual art as a medium through which to explore their values, experiences and views. In some of the students' works the underlying themes of health and illness are easily identifiable. In others they are less so, and relate more directly to the themes of the PPS domain, particularly *Health & Wellbeing*.

We have been impressed by the quality of critical reflection, empathy, and exploration of the themes of the PPS domains in many of our students' works. This published collection presents some of the pieces that we have been captivated by.

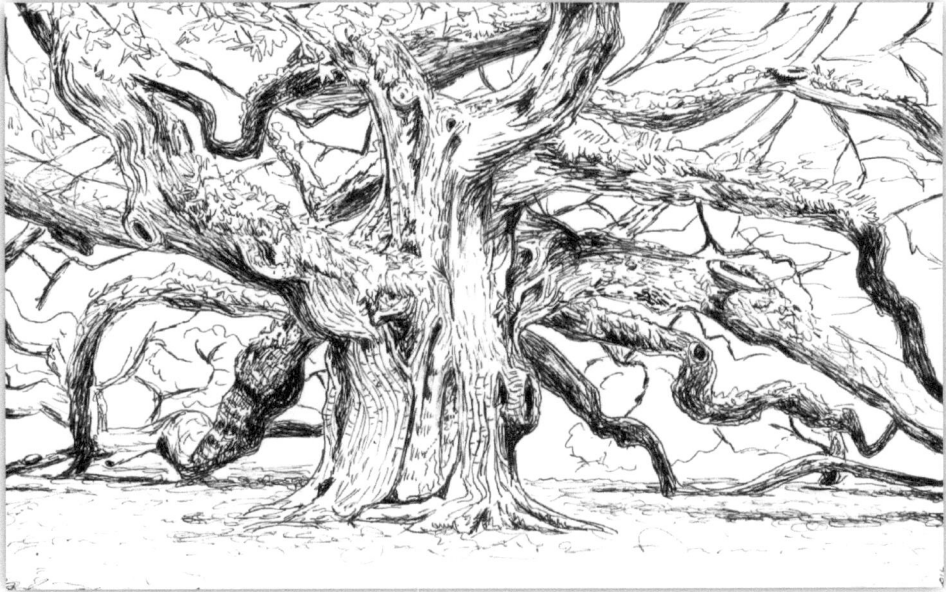

Aimee Vulinovich, Year 5, *Oaktree*. 2016. Fountain pen ink on paper. Series:
Fountain pen sketches of significant places I have visited.

The power of narrative medicine

Tanisha Jowsey and Ping Qu

"Telling stories about illness is to give voice to the body. Bodies are not just the topics of stories, but the body sets in motion the need for new stories when its disease disrupts the old stories." -Arthur Frank, 2013 (4)

Charon's seminal 2001 article (5) that introduces the idea of 'narrative medicine' begins with a gripping tale of Ms Lambert's profound sadness at the realisation that her dear son will suffer the same illness that has left her in a wheelchair; Charcot-Marie-Tooth disease. Ms Lambert explains this to her doctor. Charon quickly draws our attention to the importance of empathy in doctor-patient relationships and in clinical practices of care. The story of Ms Lambert is one of on-going suffering, tragedy, familial bonds, and chronicity. It is also one that positions the physician's subjectivities in terms of their own grief and alertness to change, inequality, and courage. Narrative medicine, which "proposes an ideal of care and provides the conceptual and practical means to strive toward that ideal" (5: 1897), begins with a physician (or indeed, any health care practitioner) reflecting on the stories that patients tell. The premise under which narrative medicine is deemed important and constructive towards better physician care of patients is that by engaging in narrative medicine the health care practitioner is encouraged to develop their sense of empathy with the patient.(5-7)

Miller and colleagues note that the intention of narrative medicine is "to provide through its pedagogy: the tools to perceive, to behold, to enter, and to represent worlds found in reality, words or pictures so as become attentive enough to effectively deliver health care to others."(8: 9) Narrative medicine also draws our attention to our own biases, stigmas, attitudes towards people, experiences, and subjectivities.(6)

During the past fifteen years we have seen an emerging body of literature concerning both narrative medicine and what Greenhalgh has termed 'narrative-based medicine.'(9, 10) This literature broadly suggests that a narrative approach to medicine is complementary with, and opposite to, the objective 'medical gaze.'

In 2004 Dasgupta and Charon presented and evaluated a short course whereby Year 2 medical students were invited to write a reflective piece about their own personal experiences of illness.(11) By writing about personal experiences medical students were encouraged to develop their self-awareness, personally and professionally. Students in the course were then invited to read one another's writing; thus offering them an opportunity to develop what Kleinman calls 'empathic witnessing,'(12) which is a form of empathy development through simply being with a patient and acknowledging where they are at (rather than being in an active state of history taking or diagnosis and care planning). Student participants in the course reportedly found it difficult to describe their personal reflections in writing, which the authors suggest may be a result of their enculturation into medicine. Students found the process of reading from their personal narrative uncomfortable; raising in them feelings of nervousness and fear about how others would interpret their experience. Yet despite these difficulties – or perhaps because the course helped students to overcome them – students evaluated the course highly. Students appreciated the "rare" opportunity "to share emotional and physical vulnerability" with one another.(11: 355) They reported that the course helped them to recognise/experience the influence of their illness experience more closely than they previously had.

Following Dasgupta and Charon's early demonstration of its value, the field of narrative medicine saw a surge in the literature.(7, 13-17) In 2011 Law's study showed that patient and doctor narratives could be used to "facilitate discussion and encourage reflection on sensitive issues" between medical students, and that this approach could usefully supplement student learning from patients.(18) More recently, Miller and colleagues reported in 2014 on evaluative findings from their large focus group narrative medicine study.(8) Medical students engaged in a semester-long lecture course of narrative medicine. Following the course 130 students participated in focus groups where demonstrated awareness of the "known features of narrative medicine – attention, representation, and affiliation – and endorsed all three as being valuable to professional identity development."(8: 1) Students reported that the course had deepened their appreciation of other people's experiences and views, and that through it they had learned not to "feel personally threatened by other opinions."(8: 9)

Our medical students' Portfolios are autobiographical, and thus vastly different from other writing exercises they engage in during medical training. Students' narratives from a first-person perspective encourage them to express their own feelings, emotion and critical thinking. Another aspect of narrative medicine is the health care practitioner as patient. The process of becoming a patient can be disorienting and health care practitioners often report feeling challenged by moving from their previously held position of power to one of reliance. Narrative medicine offers an avenue through which such power and identity tensions can be explored. Our students' works have also explored the power dynamics present between themselves as students and with teachers/consultants/senior members of their health care team.

Medical students have severe pressure from their academic work and competition, and as they move into clinical roles they are faced with occupational stress that can lead to occupational burnout.(19-22) Narrative writing provides an avenue to mitigate such stresses. When we develop narrative medicine writing routines and skills they can serve to relieve pressure, promote job satisfaction, and promote effective relationships between practitioner and patient.

These are important outcomes for students and their implications can be far reaching; not only in terms of personal and professional identity and experience, but also in terms of the way we identify subjectively with others, whether they be friends, professional colleagues, patients, informal carers, neighbours, or friends we have not yet met.

What follows is the student poetry and art collection of 2016

Professionalism

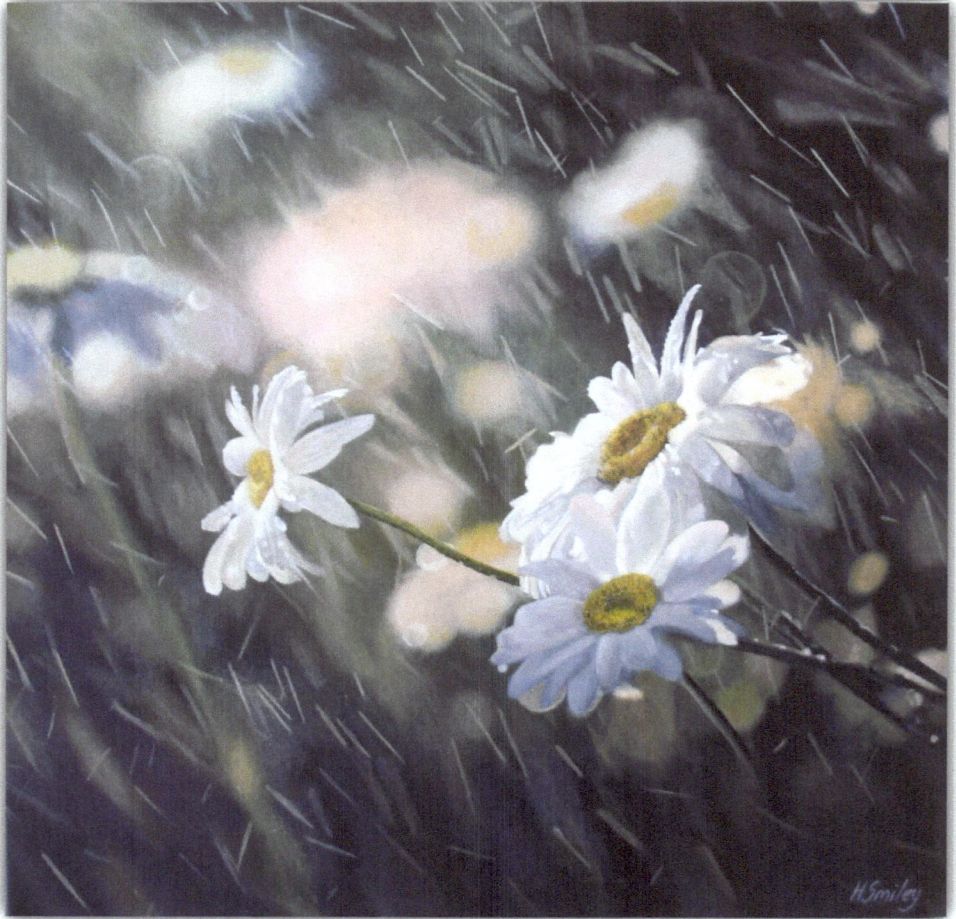

Hannah Smiley, Year 5, *Daisies*, 2016.

Learning Kindness

In primary school I learned to read, to multiply, to divide
and how to care for an egg without cracking it
I never was the best at English or math
but my egg did survive the longest
there was no award in prize giving for that
surprising because
in order to protect an egg for one week you must be thoughtful, considerate
and gentle with fragile things
but unlike reading, multiplication and division
these skills are not measured.

In medical school I have learned to measure jugular venous pressure
to prescribe fluids, to diagnose appendicitis
they like to examine these things
I have also become a holder of hands, a listener
and learned to warm my stethoscope before placing it on a chest
I have seen the importance of humor and of silence
these skills are not measured
but it is these lessons I value the most
much like how to care for an egg.

Monica Pritchard, Year 4, as Professionalism

A prayer from an 84 year old

Dear God,
I have cancer.
As I sat patiently for my clothes to dry
and for some to cease being my own
rain soaked the growing earth
and weeds spread their ruthless fingers amongst the asphodel.
I sat quietly, waiting, shivering.
But then! Those birds of yours messed my car window
Kids heaved not one but *two*
filthy tennis balls at my poor tulips.
And dear Laurie (bless his soul) who tried to make dinner,
Fell asleep while the oven cooked a dark sodden ash of passed away turnips
and cremated chicken.
So I spent the day cleaning messes and dishes and tennis balls...
God, the world ought to be a little more polite to an old woman with cancer!
But ---
just because it isn't Lord,
Praise Be to that.

Hannah Ng, Year 4, as Professionalism

Mon Beau

Beautiful baby boy
how can you smile?
How could you ever find the strength
to smile
when you never had a chance.

You came into this life without a bloody chance!

Even when you were forming
you were being poisoned
by your own Mother.
But you struggled on.

Hidden like a shameful secret.
Born in a closet
yet you persevered.

And then you tried to come out backwards
- you started to suffocate.
Half an hour you struggled
slowly dying
before anyone even called for help.

Then she left you.
Your own mother.
The one person who should always be there
to do whatever she can to help you, her son.

Furious and disgusted
I want to scream!
To cry.
I want to fight this for you.
Hold you
and hug you better.

And you smile at me as if it is *I* that needs the hug.

I pray for you little man.
Who despite all the bitterness in his innocent life
his suffering
still smiles up at me now.

Despite being deprived of love from the start
he still has enough love in himself
to give me some.
To give me an eye-crinkling, chubby-cheeked, lop-sided
Smile.

And I, born a privileged white girl
the 1% of vast opportunity;
I at times have the bloody cheek to feel self-pity.

What a joke!
No.
Be real.

We must fight for those who can't
- With no one on their side.
We owe it.

Go boy, go far.
Overcome these vicious circumstances.
Change hearts and open minds.
Touch lives.

May you have all the love you deserve
and more
all the peace of a happy healthy kid.

You have inspired me.
Hope and love for a stranger
when you had neither.
Continue to inspire us
and teach us
all to love again.

Lizzi Wilson, Year 5, as Professionalism

Creative context

This is about a beautiful baby boy I met on my Paediatrics run at Middlemore, with a tragic beginning to life that has really stuck with me. What really touched me was how those around him rallied to help give him the best chance at life, and that he had enough love in him to share it with me in a smile too.

Early morning piccolos and my lucky blue shark socks

I started out as a GP, on Dominion Road
Where the days were long and full of kids, with a runny nose
"probably a virus", I told the mums, "take Panadol, and rest."
"antibiotics," they replied. "We know our children best."
And with one member of the team refusing to get along
the first four weeks of fifth year dragged on and on and on.
Never yet in my career have I felt such apathy
it's now become quite obvious I won't be a GP.

With this done and dusted, to the hospital I moved
and while on trauma surgery my frame of mind improved.
In love with every minute, with theatre and ED
with stabbings, chest drains, trauma calls and laparotomies.
With suturing and wearing scrubs and navy Birkenstocks
with early morning piccolos and my lucky blue shark socks.

"Demi you're not indestructible and while you're very good"
you need to slow down sometimes, am I understood?"
(In my end-of-trauma-meeting), is what the consultant said,
so I took this to the extreme and did psychiatry instead.
Only kidding – given a choice I wouldn't make the switch
I think I'll always be (at heart) a high pace surgi b***h.

But I spent six weeks in forensic psych, which frequently entailed
some very interesting trips to Paremoremo Jail
and meanwhile on Mondays I do confess there's something you should know
That I always blow off study and instead watch Game of Thrones.
Good news, I think I always knew that Jon Snow wasn't dead
but I'll never forgive Joffery for removing his dad's head.
Now don't you worry, I haven't been folly and the rest of the week I'll be
Reading and learning (and dreaming and yearning of being on surgery).

This poem wouldn't be complete without thinking back on paeds,
snotty noses and cheeks like roses and kids not taking feeds.
Three broken arms and a false alarm in ED late at night
(no those are not chicken pox, just a few flea bites).
Trudging along for five-hour rounds- as redundant as redundant could be
when I realised I was being bullied, I couldn't help but think. *What? Me?*
And though people seem to think surgeons are the ones we should fear
the culprit was in fact a registrar who I avoided going near.

As the year goes on the night is long and for now I am done,
although I'll probably add some more after the end of the next run.
No apologies will be made if this has left you unimpressed
or if you are concerned about how quickly I digressed
But another year has come and gone, there's one thing I now know

it's that where your passion truly lies, that direction you should go.

So something I remember when things are getting rough
is nothing makes me happier than, quite frankly, cutting stuff.
Of course I do appreciate that it's not an easy life
but anyway, I never felt inclined to just be a good housewife.

Demi Poynter, Year 5, as Professionalism

Looking for ulcers

"It hurts so much," he breathes
peering down,
"It's been that way for months."

You forget your medication, have crumbs
on the collar of your sweater, and
croak in a smoker's voice. But
I sit at your feet and listen to what you say.

And then to examine:
unthreading the shoelaces
twisting off the heel
peeling away the socks
hitching up the trouser legs –
on one side
        and then the other.

The skin was livid, purple, stiff and cold.
My fingers press behind the ankle
as if knocking on a closed door.
No pulse responds in kind.

There, wearing low on the shin are
two sunken pits each
a muddy hole with
puckered edges like rotting craters.

Joyce Leung, Year 5, as Professionalism

Untitled

A 111 call comes in
Flashing lights and sirens begin
Tragedy at the naturist park
The tone in the ambulance, quiet and dark

We arrive to greet despair
You can feel the sombreness in the air
A resident found a deceased man
Hanging in his caravan

As we draw closer my heart doth sink
But I can handle this, or so I think
A sight to behold I shall never forget
I catch my breath, palms cold and wet

What sorrow must this man have known
To feel that he was so alone
His only option to end the strife
To make the decision to end his life

The day goes on and I'm home, it's late
I'm exhausted but can't help contemplate
The day's events uniquely intense
Processing this will be hard I sense

I call my mother in the UK
I'm not sure what I'm going to say
Before I know it I'm sobbing down the phone
"Mum, I've had such an awful day!" I moan

At 25 and though a man
With life experience and a plan
I'll never not need my family
They are my outlet, they support me

Medicine can be an exacting field
The highs and lows that we yield
Health, Disease, Life and Death
A dichotomous world from breath to breath

Josh Coulter, Year 5, as Professionalism

Creative context

During my selective rotation in the emergency department in Tauranga, I accompanied the paramedics for a shift. The following poem describes one job we received, which was to attend a suicide and attempts to convey the whirlwind of emotions I felt during and after.

View from Inside

Year 9:

He drinks from his brother's beer bottle
stealing sips when he's not looking
It feels warm and tingly trickling down his throat
he's 14 now and it's time to become a man.

Year 10:

He drinks on a Friday night to be cool
mixing bourbon with his blood.
It gives him confidence – liquid courage.

Year 11:

He drinks straight from the bottle, hard glass against cold teeth
seeping into his veins and navigating familiar streets to his brain.
Drowning in intoxication with no one there to pull him out.
Passing out on the bedroom floor...
He'll stay there until morning.

Year 12:

He drinks to forget;
the ringing in his ears
the bruises that he wears
the father that he fears.

Year 13:

He drinks until he's angry
stalking the streets looking for someone to fight;
breath staggers out of him, irregular white puffs in the night.
Knuckles meet bone and the taste of iron fills his mouth
he tumbles to the ground, face pressed into the gravel
arms wrenched behind his back and metal cuffs wrapped around his wrists.
He's 18 now, and he's been trapped for years.

Will Utley, Year 5, as Professionalism

Life

Some say life is
From the magical moment of conception.
The gift from above,
The mystery of a new beginning.
A being whose sanctity is paramount.

Some say life is
The right for a woman to choose.
Her body is her own,
A potential vessel for a future generation
But only when she is ready.

Some say life is
The processes your cells undergo.
The anatomical framework of your bones,
Muscles, tongue and eyes.
A fleshy organism with the mental capacity to judge.

Some say life is
The belonging of a greater being.
That one is a vessel
Of something much greater,
A reflection of another world on Earth.

Some say life is
Being able to succeed.
Running and swimming your way
Through triumphs at work and home.
Nothing can stop your ability to think freely.

Some say life is
Not just what one can or can't do.
Disability and disease
Don't take away from who you are.
A wheelchair can't put restraints upon your spirit.

Some say life is
Living inside reality.
If you can't see straight,
Or recognise the ones you love,
There is no point in existing.

Some say life is
Until the very end.

When you take your last breath
And your hands go cold.
When your soul flees this plane of existence.

Some say life is
Who you are.
How you write your path
And the decisions you make.
Life could just be .... you.

Tom Doolin, Year 5, as Professionalism

Creative context

This poem captures the many different perspectives on the meaning of life that a medical student comes across in the hospital. It reflects on how you have to take these varying world views into account in the clinical setting.

Treat yourself: a poem about patient stereotypes in medicine

If I were a teenage mother of three
Who barely scrapes to make end meets
Or a pregnant lawyer who has
Taken all the recommended vitamins
And done exactly what you want.
Would you treat me the same?

If I were that homeless rugged fellow
Who always bothers you about change
Or the charming, intelligent son
Of your fellow orthopaedic surgeon.
Would you treat me the same?

If I were a stoic, Maori chain-smoker
Who refused to quit for the fifth time
Or a blonde Remuera housewife
Who you have seen in private.
Would you treat me the same?

If I were the scrawny drug addict
Who had just been diagnosed with HIV
Or the social, young engineer
Who has come for relief of her joint.
Would you treat me the same?

If I were the man who's a bit slow
Going for surgery with a BMI of 45
Or the sister of your best mate
Who keeps fit at the gym.
Would you treat me the same?

If I were the lady of oriental extraction
Who cannot understand a word you say
Or the woman who brought you into this world
Who understands without you saying a word.
Would you treat me the same?

If I were the borderline girl
Who you've seen five times for self-harm
Or the woman who brings you baking
And has come for relief of her sniffles.
Would you treat me the same?

If you were the doctor who judged each patient
Like the cover of a book
Or the doctor who treated patients
For the individuals they are
With empathy and understanding.
Would you treat yourself the same?

Tom Doolin, Year 5, as Professionalism

Creative context

The inspiration for the poem are stereotypes that doctors attach to patients that can result in differential treatment. It highlights the efforts we must go to as medical practitioners to not judge others and to make sure that patients do not feel stigmatised by their differences.

Cancer's Plight

ED by night
Screaming drunkard two curtains away
my mother praying as she soothes my grandma's blown up
belly
in a circular motion
A rough rub of a weathered hand on coarse uniform fabric
It hurts, it hurts
Blinding bed light, necessary
for doctor to place icy hands on distended abdomen
four tender quadrants, negative murphy's
bowels not moving
Of course it's not, it's the cancer Doc
It's the cancer in the belly
and the cancer in the kidneys, the pelvis, the lymph nodes
the brain
Let me die, let me die

It is no different at home
mouth dry, like it's been filled with
sand
we try to wash it out with hot tea, cold juice, Listerine
but the grains are stubborn
they smother the taste buds
eating is but a mere task
one of the few tasks now, unless you count lying in bed
with intermittent fevers, hot and cold sweats, peaking
at 2am
A rainbow of pills three times a day with meals, please
it's just placebo
hair still shedding, bones still aching
Is this life worth living?
Why yes
for what is beyond death?
I want to see my grandchildren married, I can't do that
where I am going
The final task is acceptance
But how, but why
stop asking me to let go of
this glorious life
Let me live, let me live

Ruyan Chen, Year 4, as Professionalism

Psychiatry in Threes

Psychiatry is hard.
Patients are troubled.
Kids aren't carefree.
Girls get worried.
Boys break things.
No one understands them.
Everyone's been hurt.
Will they recover?
I'm not sure.

One girl arrives.
She is sixteen.
She is quiet.
Her dad died.
She hasn't grieved.
She stays closed.
Questions bother her.
One word answers.
The air's heavy.
The silence hurts.
She fidgets away.
The hour's up.
She practically runs.
Mum is helpless.
She's tried everything.
What is next?

One boy arrives.
He is fifteen.
He likes stealing.
He likes porn.
He lights fires.
The police know.
Home is hard.
Fights happen lots.
Dad is furious.
Mum's fed up.
She's tried everything.
They're foster parents.
He loves them.
He feels remorse.
But porn's fun.
Stealing is fun.
Rules are silly.

So it goes.
Over and over.
Day after day.
Girl after boy.
It saddens me.
And worries me.

Psychiatry is hard.
But it's common.
They need help.
Do doctors help?
Do drugs help?
I'm not sure.

Steva Rumsey, Year 5, as Professionalism

Stepping Stone

Your stepping stones have
not yet been embedded into
this concrete ground
but do not look down, for we
need you with us now

Know that you are still warm
your golden coat glistening
bake them the armour
our hands no longer burn

Know that you are still pure
your blood still transparent
pour your heart into the gaps
our hollow stethoscopes
leave behind

Know that when we become
blind, we use your eyes
when our heels wear off,
your footprints remain
when our hands stay
cold, we rely on the touch
that we do not own

Medical student
Know that you are useful.
Know that you can help.
Know that we need you.

Welcome to the team.

Gerald Lee, Year 5, as Professionalism

Dr. Hitler

Morning all, what a good day
Hold on, in my office now Nate!
Did I say you don't need to wear a tie?
Now you've made me mad, and it's only eight

What happened overnight?
Excuse me, you don't know?
Mr Perrett with the Cushing's,
Which idiot referred him to Ortho?

Mr Reidy with the pancreatitis
He could have become septic
Tell me you at least know
What to do when a patient becomes hypoglycaemic

Don't just stand there like a dork
What use is that going to do?
Answer me, what do you do for nec fasc!
Even the fourth year knows more than you

Oh, you're quaking in your boots now
I'll let you enjoy my wrath
My passive aggressiveness
Shows you're walking a treacherous path

Why, that's put a leap in my step
Let us go to our next consult
Who'll be the victim this time?
I have no problem pointing out all your faults
Patient, take off your top!
Come on don't be shy
Our students need to learn
There's no need to cry

Ruyan Chen, Year 4, as Professionalism

Edward

Why do you hate me, can you not love more of me?
Why does everything change when there's another chromosome you see?

I may not have a palette, but I promise my heart is pure
my ears may be low set, how I wish there was a cure

My chromosomes they cheated me
this isn't something I can choose
but I'm the one who has to pay
please let this be a rouse

Kaveshan Naidoo, Year 5, as Professionalism

The Motive

Passion or prestige, motives for degrees,
We call it nobility, is everything as it seems?

A false sense of security
can we really call that esteem?

In a profession of a routine
is there any space to dream?

They call it saving lives,
but is that really what they mean?

When in reality it's a scheme
of egos and bursting seams

Politics that can't be calmed with a soothing cream.

Kaveshan Naidoo, Year 5, as Professionalism

Public Health

Hauora Māori, we are taught
Te Whare Tapu Wha;
We need all to be well.
Taha Tinana, physical
Taha wairua, spiritual
Taha whānau, family
Taha hinengaro, mental.

But we are missing you,
Aku tamariki, my children
Oku teina, oku tuaine, my brothers and sisters
Our siloed health system
Inadequate to meet your needs.

If we focus on one area
But the others are mauiui
You cannot get better
We are not fixing the problem;
Time and money ineffectively spent

For if we are attempting to address your physical health,
Yet your home is a drafty garage
Your walls are mouldy
Your floor is cold concrete
How will you get better?

If we are attempting to address your mental health,
But you feel no connectivity to your land,
Your iwi,
Your whanau,
Your purpose
Your Mauri and mana ake,
How will you get better?

If we are attempting to address your whānau's material needs
But grandma is sick in hospital,
Brother has dropped out of school
Mum sleeps all day and won't get up in the mornings
And little sister has a leaky heart valve
How have we really helped?

We are the service industry,
Servant leaders,
Not paternalistic preachers
What service are we really providing?

Doctors, Nurses, Physios
Social workers, Psychologists and Teachers
Social Welfare and housing
Names and Titles
Walls and Buildings

Divided funding systems

Why are we split up
Blaming one another
And working separately
On the same bigger problem;
Like children who refuse
To play nicely together.

We cast our nets wide
To catch the fish
Swimming in difficult seas
But we miss those
Who need us most.

Disparity gaps spread
Like white light through a prism
We are all human
But do not live the same.

One mother, One father
One land,
Many people

Rise up! tē whanau,
Nga hapu
Te hapori
Te iwi

And you!
Providers and leaders
Agencies and practices

Come together! I say
Take a stand!
Mau ringa
Kia kaha
Let servant join servant
And give all we have;
Time and money
Love and compassion
Understanding and empathy

Take from us; the wealthy
and give to our deprived
whose voices have gone unheard too long
This ends with us.

Lizzi Wilson, Year 5, as Professionalism

I Met a Man Today

I met a man today.

He is old and I am young.
He is dying, I am well.

He is lost.
So am I.

I met a man today.

I held his hand, I felt his pain.

Tears roll down his writhing, broken body. Screams of anguish, confusion, desperation.

His body fighting, his eyes empty. Part of him already gone.
His body missed the memo.

He gasps for breath, body shaking. His arm snaps outwards, a pale blur.
My arm exposed, fingers squeezing, nails sinking deep

His strength takes my breath.
One last try. I can see it in his face. Why will she not help me?

The sharpness of the pain feels odd, far away, detached.
The heavy aching in my chest does not.

My words of comfort comfort no one.

I met a man today.

It was not peaceful, it was not quick.

His family gone. His nurse too busy.

Just sit with him until he passes. Then come and join us on the ward round.

Anonymous, as Professionalism

The 96y/old male in Room 1C

You sit before me
And the cold, clinical room disappears as I pull back
The canary yellow curtains
Their patterned cloth giving us the illusion of privacy
As the body next door continues to splutter

You sit before me,
And smooth out your sheets
Your wizened hands and tired soul
Not yet ready to let go of dignity
Not yet ready to admit you are old

You sit before me,
And you speak of your cough
We speak about your family
We speak about the war,
The wrinkles in your eyes concealing secrets
Ninety-six years in the making

You sit before me
You talk about going home soon
And we laugh about the weeds in your vege garden
The reality of your condition hangs in the air
An unspoken truth we both dance around
A beautiful ballet

You sit before me
You are tired and pale
Not strong enough to fight
But not quite ready to let go
Not quite ready to admit you are old

You sit before me
And watch young students scurry on in their lives
So wrapped in the certainty of youth
I wonder what you used to look like
Before age touched your skin and your soul

I don't know what happened to you
Whether you made it home or not
And I never got to tell you
What a privilege it was
To have you sit before me

Emily Aitken, 2015, Year 4, as Professionalism

The Geriatric Experience

Walking through the ward
Through open doors I sometimes see
People in a state, I don't think
They ever wished to be

Blank eyes, open mouths
Trained on the bleak wall
I cannot help but think
Are they looking at their pall?

Being but a shadow
Of what they used to be
Despair and pity
Overcome me

Yet
When beside them in a chair
The realisation dawns upon me
They are still there

Despite their diminishing senses
Amidst the mental scree
Their humanity triumphantly emerges
Plain for all to see

They may not understand
Everything I say
But I don't mind when they speak
To me of their hey-day

Or a time remembered with fondness
Reminds me of why I am here
To care for people regardless
If parts of them disappear

Saiprasad Ravi, Year 4, as Professionalism

It's an Emergency.

Vulnerable. Exposed.
It's like being a part of another world lying there on the operating bed.
Time out, they say. Any concerns?
It's an emergency.

There was no mention that her baby might die,
but her face said it all, looking into her eyes you could see the unknown...
the fear... the terror...
It's an emergency.

But who had time to notice her eyes?
I did.
Who had time to hold her hand?
I did.
Who had time to talk her through?
I did.
That's all part of being a medical student in an emergency.

Anonymous, as Professionalism

Creative context

On my Obstetrics & Gynaecology placement I attended an emergency caesarean section and it was looking like a poor prognosis for the baby. With a spinal anaesthetic in place the patient was awake and terrified. Not having an essential role as part of the medical team, I took the time to comfort and support her in a terrifying and unfamiliar situation – an essential role as a medical student.

A long night

It was the longest night that one
Stretched out over two blue hospital chairs
Each promising a comfort they could not provide
Watching monitors and flashing lights
Aware of each breath you made

The whorl of your silver hair cushioned your head
Your hand sat atop a pillow, tucked safely into mine
With its tissue-thin skin revealing bruise after bruise
Each symbolising a different trauma
A different battle we had all overcome

I soon realised the true value of the hospital cannulator
The euphoria of seeing her walking through the door
Knowing your little veins would be saved from damage
Your little body saved from unnecessary pain
Our hearts saved from having to watch you go through it

Clean gowns, cups of tea, linen changes,
All these things impacted our journey so much more
Than the constant passage of Doctors that graced the room
Ten minutes a day, another patient on the list
Words spoken over us, to us, about you, to you

Many people think their Grandma is the most amazing thing in the world
But they are wrong; because mine actually is
My Grandma is a fizzing cracker-wazzoom jacker-Sequin stacker
Celery snacker-life attacker
Most wonderful-sassy-stylish-spontaneous person I know

Until one day, life popped her bubble of fizz
So two surgeries, three months of hospital, four visiting specialist
Five bags of blood, six courses of antibiotics and <u>countless</u> hospital meals later
Here you were; low blood pressure, high temperature. Exhausted
So our journey began of the longest night

"Best to have that conversation" the surgeon said
As you balanced perilously on life's gossamer thread
Denial, panic, fear, desperation washed over me
Like the tidal wave of medical jargon that came afterwards
Relentless, and rigid.

And while frantic phone calls were made
In dark and sleepy hospital corridors
I sat with you, watching you sleep
Counting your breathing
Waiting for the next nursing visit

Would you be lying here if it weren't for me?
Would we have done the surgery if I didn't say it was for the best?
Thought after thought rushed through me

And the panic of feeling personally responsible crashed over me,
A leaden weight, in the pit of my stomach

I know you would be horrified to know
How I sat there thinking
Of how stupid I was to think I knew how this would go
To think I knew what was best for you
Just a stupid girl, with stupid thoughts who doesn't know her own limits.

And as each insecurity of mine reared its ugly head
The minutes slipped by gently and quietly
Turning into hours that beckoned the sun
The hospital starting to hum again with noise
The darkness was banished to its scary corner

You pulled through in the end
"Saw the other side and didn't like it"
Was your comment I think
"Plus we never made those cushions"
"Tell your dad I'll be at the beach house this summer."

Anonymous, as Professionalism

Creative context
This year my grandmother, who I am very close to, ended up hospitalized for three months. During this time, I learnt from personal perspective what truly makes a good doctor and what actually matters when you are walking through a difficult time in hospital with your loved one. This poem, entitled "A long night" describes the night I was left alone in my thoughts by her bedside when we came very close to losing her after a major surgery.

Breaking
Lettuce in his teeth
filling the void
between the second and third teeth.

It fluttered, slightly,
with every emph-flutter-urable word.
C-flutter-ancer. Inc-flutter-urable. Ch-flutter-emotherapy.
... or maybe it was just the C-words
that c-flutter-aused the tremulous green wave

Really, it spoiled any chance
the patently affected sympathy had.

I don't blame him, not really
I mean he had, like
his whole long life still to live,
being important, telling people about
30% survival rates and stage 3 invasion.

He was about to launch such a campaign
against my very own invasion;
and I mean, couldn't I really do more
than simply lie back and take the news?!

His vaguely stifled sigh
-I wish you'd hurry up and start crying
so I can leave you with the nurses -
set the green flag thrashing.

I willed it free
to add another comedic element
to the farce of my breaking.
Breaking of news, breaking of body;
they seem to be one and the same?

Green go ahead on the news of my impending death.

Allie Rout, Year 5, as Professionalism

Psychosis Flower

What is psychosis
but a flower
that grows in the fields of our minds.

Nurtured by hail and thunder
it grows in stormy weather
roots snake deeper
forming cracks
in our framework.

It can be bold and bright
A wildflower
a sight to behold
petals of red and yellow, pink and blue and orange and green and
fluoroandleopardprint…

Or it can be small and black.
Grey.
Bleak.
Mottled blue and cold.
Still and quiet and menacing.
Feeding off our life force…
Draining us.
Twisted vines bind us tight
trapped by our own feelings and thoughts.

As its roots spread
It reaches our ears
And we gain unwanted friends;
whispering, whispering.
It reaches our eyes,
painting patterns on the walls
visions of dreams and nightmares.
Butterflies flutter and demons crawl.

You promise improvements and side effects
but I do not want your pills and potions.
Your jabs and stabs.
That killer for the weeds in my mind
makes me sick too
fat and sleepy.
Jerky and restless.
How can I explain,
Doctor,
when my thoughts are not my thoughts
someone tosses them like a salad.
My tongue is not my tongue
angels and demons play tug-of-war
with my words
and my brain is a desert
parched of sleep.

My mood is a yo-yo.
My energy an empty well.
My motivation a straight-jacket.
For fun I watch my thoughts play cat-and-mouse
and sleep evades me still.

And all the while
my bewitching flower grows
Ensnaring my mind.
I am trapped
in a world very different to yours.
Whose is real?

Lizzi Wilson, Year 5, as Professionalism

Creative context

These two pieces (Psychosis Flower and Schizophrenia Diagnosis) were inspired by some of the people I met on my psychiatry run in Otahuhu Community Mental Health, as well as by someone close to me, and the ways they opened my eyes to their perspective on life and reality and made me question – is what we are doing really right?

Schizophrenia Diagnosis

You and me, my friend
we'll be together forever.
Every minute of every day.
No more privacy
no more quiet
no more alone.
I have your peace
I have your thoughts.
Try run, go on.
Every room you ever go in
I'll already be there
waiting.
and it's not just you
I can get to them too
You'll be struggling against me
forever and ever
until the end of time.

They know now too
vivid in your folder by your name
screaming black
like a tattoo
etched deep in your skin
but the ink seeps deeper.

Burns your mind
mind's eye
minds fly
fly, fly away!
Be free,
free as a bee
buzzy bee
busy bee
busy buzzyness
busyness
business
as a registered bee inspector
eye wink to ewe
chuckle
Huckleberry Finn
Steinback and friends...
Voluminous.
Peace story to you.

Lizzi Wilson, Year 5, as Professionalism

Intimate Partner Violence
(20th June 2016)

Intimate partner violence.
A term that should not be shrouded in silence.
For too long it has been such.
A personal problem between a husband and wife.
Behind closed doors, so far removed from everyday life.

A taboo, to not be indulged or explored.
Where a black eye and bruises are simply "I tripped and I fell."
Where everything is controlled and 'control' is everything;
From the people you speak to, to the time outside the door.
An entire life filled with excuses, to the outside that doesn't want to know more.

It spans all races and classes,
Not just the poor and impoverished.
And it may seem easier to simply turn a blind eye,
But this is a world where there are families and friends,
At times faced with the question, just when will this burden end?

Intimate partner violence.
A term now not so shrouded in silence.
For now times are changing and you can get help.
The great ol' television instructs that "It's Not Okay."
You see billboard after billboard on your way home,
There are ribbons galore,
White for sexual abuse against women,
Purple for domestic abuse,
Even blue for abuse against our children.

We have wondrous agencies.
Many fight day after day to change the landscape,
To re-craft society into a place where this is not accepted,
Where victims can reach out, get help and change their future.
This is what they make their mandate!
Where abuse is not welcome,
Not in any shape or form.
Where the very society that used to turn their heads,
Now shake them vigorously in disapproval.
A wholesome society where people are equal,
And there are no queries of 'control.'
Where victims can say no and
remove themselves from this endless spiral.

Where they can grow, move on and thrive.
Where abusers, condemned with shame and guilt,
Can learn skills and ideas to re-integrate and survive.

Intimate partner violence.
A term we hope to remove from silence.
But what does this mean for me?
Fighting for justice and equality.
It means more than just verbal support.
How can it be deemed enough for me to say
simply, I support you and all you've done today
but not ask the hard questions about abuse and violence?

As a student
I mustn't take it lightly for It happens too often.
And when 1 in 3 women have experienced it,
More time on my hands may be just what is needed.
For all that is needed is to ask.
To start a conversation, and hear their story,
Maybe all that is needed to change their trajectory.

As a future doctor,
It means I must support the system.
Support each and every cog,
From the screening questions to the ribbons
the multiple agencies to new initiatives.
Initiatives that go by population health approaches.
Especially one which thinks of the big picture, the upstream approach.

For the future this means
being open to new ideas
listening to people
striving to develop viable solutions
and working to create a just system.
One which won't fail, like it failed those who suffer today.
One that will be there in the first instance
to act as a safety net, as a preventative measure.
One that caters for all races and classes
and serves not to penalise, but change society itself.
A system that grows and changes with time.
A system I hope to help change over time.

And so, intimate partner violence.
It's a term that I hope to help remove from silence.

Nikhil Magan, Year 5, as Professionalism

Creative context
This poem is an expression of some of the ideas I encountered during our Population Health Intensive week, where we were at times confronted with some difficult stories of intimate partner violence as we strived to develop a suitable public health strategy to tackle this major problem as part of our brief for the project.

Time Management

I studied so much through the day
I did not take the time to play.

When people said, "come out with me"
I told them "not now," and quietly

I continued on, feeling crook
trying to read every textbook.

When people said "take time for you"
I'd say, "I have too much to do."

But then it seems "I saw the light."
An end came to my sorry plight.

By better managing my time
I now fully enjoy my prime

Life's too short not to socialise
I just need to prioritise.

I take the time to go and do
all the things that I'm wanting to.

I'm happy and relaxed at last
All-day study is in the past.

Hannah Smiley, Year 5, as Professionalism

If I were a Patient Today

If I were a patient today
What a different world it would be
To be unaware of my room, neighbours and procedures,
To be unable to control my routine, meal times and sleep patterns,
To put my regular life on hold for a period of time I do not know.

If I were a patient today
What would make my stay better
I would appreciate any kindness and care
I would want my care to be managed with my interests taken into account
I would hope that I meant more than a name on a piece of paper

If I were a patient today
How would I know what to ask or be aware of
If I was flicked around between different teams and specialties
If I was caught in the middle of an argument between two doctors
If I was talked over and could never ask a question

If I were a patient today
How can I rest
Not knowing who would come and examine me next
Not knowing what stereotypes were being made behind my back
Not knowing why I was being poked and prodded by different machines

If I were a patient today
I would want my doctor to know
I can hear the mutters you say under their breath about me and other patients
I can see the dreaded look you have as you enter my room every morning
I can feel that I am a burden on your already busy day

I know that my discharge would mean one less patient and an easier day
I know you may think I am making symptoms up but I would rather not be in
hospital either
I know that there are people sicker than me but I would still appreciate compassion
sometimes
I know you tell me what is going on but I cannot remember everything to tell my
family
I know I have a condition but I am more than that one thing I promise you

I know all this
You do not need to remind me of it
Even though you may not say it
Or write it
I know all about it

Anonymous, as Professionalism

It's Not Okay

It's okay, I'm used to it

The forced smile practiced a thousand times
Eagerly waiting for the time to pass
Eyes shut tight wishing it was a dream
Why are you being treated like this

It's okay, I'm used to it

Patches and blotches that cover your skin
One or two times won't make something like this
Seven years has been far too long
Why do you not cry or say that it's wrong

It's okay, I'm used to it

I'm used to it... words never to be learnt
A family loving and caring is what you deserve
Love and support to help you grow
But why is it you are always alone

It's okay, I'm used to it

Who can imagine the pain you've been through
Living ignorant but still complaining
Sorry you have been so ignored
No longer will you be left alone

It's not okay

Daniel Lee, Year 5, as Professionalism

I.C.U*

I sometimes feel this loneliness
Like the ache of an old infection.

Sometime I can forget about it
Subsumed amongst the regular
Modicum of Being.

Roar, Roar, Roar
And like a fire it burns
Into the ashes
Of my soul.

My parchment is dry
And the script that engenders the
Story of my life
Have no words but the harsh
Crags of emptiness.

I sought a God, and
Amongst the darkness, I found
A single, shivering flower illuminated
By flickering candlelight.

Burn, Burn, Burn
And into the darkness I cried
And I cried.

For what shall go out
If not the light, but then the soul?

Anonymous C., as Professionalism

Creative context

Studying medicine can be challenging. Sometimes, we experience situations that make us feel alone. Upon occasion, we witness stories that drive us to ponder over some of life's greatest mysteries.

*ICU: Intensive Care Unit

Ethics and the Law

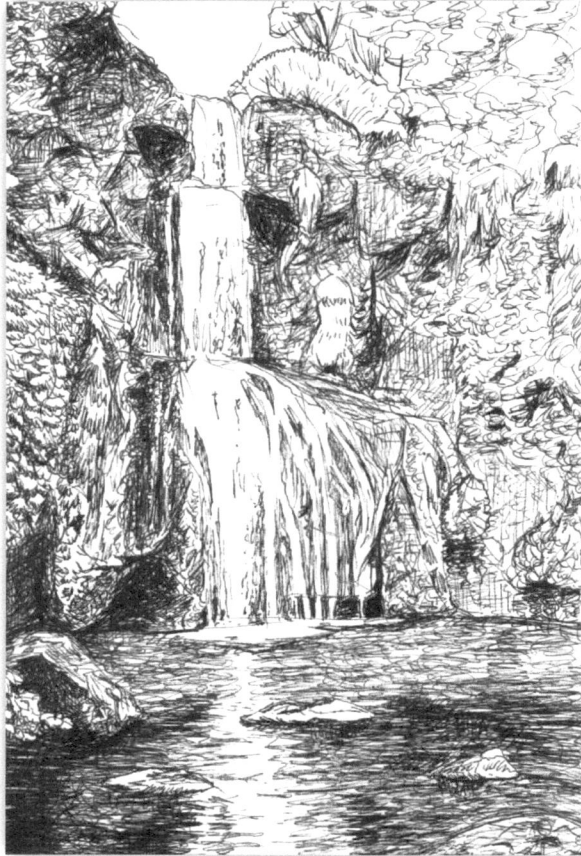

Aimee Vulinovich, Year 5, *Kite Kite Falls, Piha.* 2016. Fountain pen ink on paper.
Series: Fountain pen sketches of significant places I have visited.

Gender

I see the women around me fighting for respect
I am yelled at on the street
I hear women discussed like objects
I wonder why the doctors in the hospital and my male peers comment on my appearance
I never comment on theirs
I am called aggressive and uncouth for behaving as the boys do
I am told that if I acted more feminine it would be easier to get a boyfriend
I am told that I should reconsider surgery as a career, because one day I will want lots of kids
I watch strangers look women up and down
I hear boys discuss what they think different women would be like in bed

I read that one in three of Auckland University's female students will be sexually assaulted
I hear the boys say that women make it up, for revenge or self-preservation
I see the media report a rapist's sporting achievements
I read a news article titled 'she said no, but did she really mean it?'
I hear a lawyer compare saying you are on the pill with consent
I am told to be careful, and take care of my friends on nights out
I hear the boys I know make rape jokes
I feel scared for us

I hear the boys I know proudly proclaim they are not feminists, because they believe in equality
I try to explain that feminism is about equality; but at this point, after centuries of oppression and violence, it will first take equity
I am called argumentative and opinionated
I feel exasperated

How can I show them what it is like to be valued based on appearance, even in a professional environment? To be treated as less capable because of my gender?
How can I make them understand what it is like to feel scared of an entire gender? That the threat of violence is a constant consideration whenever we do anything, wear anything, or drink anything?
How can I make them understand when they won't even listen to my voice?

Anonymous, as Ethics & The Law

PR Examination Under Anaesthesia*

No formal introduction
No awkward conversation
No getting into position
There was no consent

The Dr told us you had already consented
But how?
The Dr did not know that we would be coming to theatre that day
It was day one

I think he may have said it to 'cover his bases'
As our faces twisted uneasily when he instructed us to do it

So limp
So lifeless
No resistance
Already asleep

He was here for surgery on his bladder
He would not have expected this

My fingers were too short
I felt nervous and uncomfortable
I could hardly feel a thing
Let alone a prostate
What a waste

This sick feeling
The unethical situation
A patient taken advantage of
For nothing

Never again
Not in any circumstance
I would rather be sent out of theatre
Than do it again

Anonymous, as Ethics & the Law

*PR: per rectal

Cancer - The Calamitous Infection

Footsteps shuffle, curtains draw
Pen in paper, faces drawn tight- austere.
Men and women gather, around the bed
Like navel officers, ready, braced and brimming.
With one commander, one captain they follow.
Small in stature but large in might, the captain leads
Troops march into battle, to conquer, to vanquish.
Like the Napoleon of medicine, he appears,
ready to fight.

But unlike Napoleon, enemy troops were not his fear
Much more formidable was his opponent,
a track record of 100-none, seemingly unconquerable.
A long fight, yes it has been; the mystery of this enemy,
hidden in the midst of fear and the unknown.
Emerging to take all there is to know.
Frustratingly, the enemy is oneself,
and its refusal to behave, like detractors from a republic
wrecking havoc from within.

Gaunt and haggard he appeared,
like a weary soldier after years of strife.
However, unlike the commander reporting back to his post,
There is no Churchill bestowing a medal of honour,
there is no foreseeable end to this war.
The only certitude worthy of derivation
Is death itself.

Napoleon and his troops align,
ready, poised to deliver the news.
Unbeknownst to him, his troops despised what was about to be done.
It was reckless, unscrupulous and dishonourable,
a disgrace to our vocation; undermining the integrity of our cause.
Regardless, words flew, knees buckled and the truth hit, square.

Yellow, itching and fatigued,
with scratch marks laden on his skin,
a tear of desolation rolling down his cachexic cheek.
Emotions flood, plunging deep into the torrential waters.
Confusion, fear, uncertainty, hopelessness, dejection.
Mouths were moving.

Sound waves compressing and refracting.
But he could not hear.

Hamish Wu, Year 4, as Ethics & The Law

Creative context
This poem describes the breaking of bad news to a patient who had a pancreatic mass which was later identified as a tumour. The breaking of bad news made me feel uncomfortable. There was little compassion in doing so.

I know it, you know it, but she doesn't.

Never in my life have I felt more like a wolf hiding.
Masking myself in a sheep's skin.
Never in my life have I questioned my morals so.
Never have I ever smiled a smile so grim.
The knife in her back, did it come from my hands?
I stare at her.
Look her dead in the eye and smile.
If I don't smile she will know.
I know it.
He knows it.
We all know it.
Cancer we said.
Palliative we said.
But we just smile sweetly and send her home.
We have to wait for the smoking gun.
The facts.
The proof.
The evidence.
We all know it.
There is a reaper in the corner.
And everyone sees it.
Everyone but her.
It's coming.
Edging its way closer.
Do I warn her.
There is a monster in her room.
There is a black cloud following her.
Its out for her.
No one can stop it.
Do I warn her.
Let her worry.
Or do I just smile.
While the reaper smiles its sick and twisted smile at me.
Its playing a game with me.
And I know how it ends.
Me and her.
We both lose.

Sandi Reweti, Year 4, as Ethics & The Law

Consonants, vowels and lost sounds

Please doctor, please,
Just because you string the letter twice together
Bring down the lines between your eyes
To give power to your mouth.
Just because your words escape you on
A sigh you can't keep trapped,
I don't understand your words. Aue?

'Aue eaeaio o oieai,'

You play notes along her spine
And she coughs out the vibrations.
Crackles and drags on notes I once
Knew as tiny whispers that wove her dreams.
You look at me like you aren't sure
How she made it eleven young years
Because she's bone-white and shaking.

'Aue eaeaio o oieai,'

But I know her as a tiny atomic bomb;
Boundless energy bled into my veins,
thread back to my heart.
Once I cut myself in our garden
While she wept; I thought I'd cleaned it all
But later it was red and hot to touch.
I fear I'll feel her long after she's flat
and white against these sheets.

'Aue eaeaio o oieai, o-i-e-a-i'

You glanced at your watch.
Thrice now; are we counting down?
I took her once to watch the fireworks.
I felt bad because she was only 6 and all the books
Say to do it right tuck her in early night
But you should have seen her face
When the sky lit that midnight.

'Aue eaeaio o oieai!'

It took her years to get her mind to understand
The 'c' could be anything other than harsh and unbending
That it could be certain, innocent, mercy.
I think she loved the hard ones too much to look elsewhere
Christmas, crackers, carnivals.
Maybe that's what happened to you?
You forgot what it was to have soft words to whisper.

T J Mitchell, Year 5, as Ethics & The Law

Cultural Competence

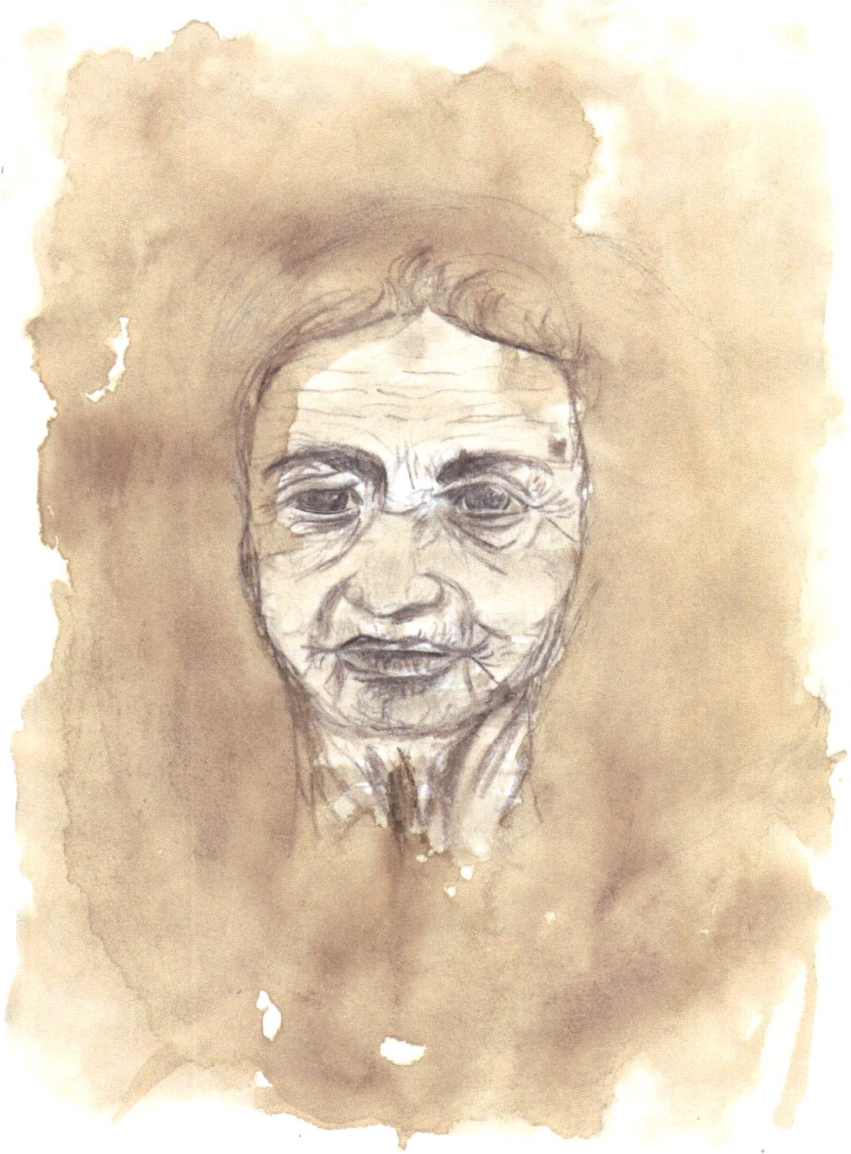

Freya Forstner, Year 4, *Whia*. 2016. Mixed media sketch.

My home visit

In our land, our people stand proud
Our women stand tall
Our men stand strong
One woman sits, her bones frail, her muscles decaying
Her face sunken with aged beauty
Cinnamon eyes hidden away behind closed curtains

She wakes with a sigh, sorrow on her breath
Heat trapped among her wardrobe of layers
Hiding her parched skin
Lips rough and worn press to my cheek as I lean in
Her breath stirs in my ears
The struggle for air commences
I count 20 breaths per minute, no 25

Her Tamāhine with water worn make up
Defeated
Her mind occupied, lost, despaired
We listen to her sobs
Her heartache becomes mine
Whanaungatanga

Our Kaumātua weeps softly
Her tamariki have kept her in their home
Nurtured and protected her
But age is winning the battle
Her cough resonates through the walls
Interrupting her lungs rhythm

Placing my stethoscope over her arched back
Her inspirations set alight sparklers through her lungs
The expirations short, almost unnoticed
Her heart ticking, out of pace
Sporadically it jumps only to return to inconsistency

Her legs fluid filled with red patches of scales
Weight bearing for only minutes
Before they ache and go weak
Functionality barely present
A wheelchair waits patiently in the garage
For its chance in the limelight

The story is harsh
Hardship and Difficulty enter the mix
Responsibility becomes the word on everyone's tongue
The whanaunga have waged warfare
For several years they've victoried
But the assault has been unsuccessful these last few months

Immobility, Illness, Infection
The cycle continues to be unbreakable

Each time the army is battered further
Stuck, lost for options, defeated
That's why we're here
To fortify the defence

One hour passes by
Our Kaumātua amongst the settled air states Rest Home
The burden in everyone reduces
A decision has finally been made
Tears of gratitude are shared
Preparations are commenced, questions are answered
We leave

In our land, our people stand proud
Our women stand tall
Our men stand strong
One woman sits, her mind made, her tears shed
Her face smiling with aged beauty
Cinnamon eyes content with what will come

Shay Richardson, Year 4, as Cultural Competence

Cultural Competence

When we met in the waiting room
No words escaped your lips as you sat and nodded
yes Doctor.
I do the talking while you smile
mutely.

It's a good prognosis I begin, thumbs up for him to know---
Okay you say, yes good
Your voice is stilted, flat as the desert plains.

And then! You spot another doctor across the way
Out comes a different tongue
As light as it is musical
Champagne
you blossom
into a fountain of sound.

Hannah Ng, Year 4, as Cultural Competence

Territory

I am a man.
I once knew my land and
It knew me.
Today we hurtle our cries into the
Emptiness.

You have made us wilder people and
as we dig through the dirt of our history
red ochre mixes with the tinge of blood that now
colours this arid paradise.

How can we begin to end what we have begun?
We sing our songs, and our songs are still to be sung.

Carmen Chan, Year 5, as Cultural Competence

Creative context

Written following a particularly memorable night shift after working with a number of Indigenous Australians presenting with conditions that had arisen as a consequence of significant health inequality.

DO NOT RESUSCITATE

(Doctor says)
Sir, you are dying
prayers cannot not save you now
miracles are merely fairytales told in church
giving false hope
to the weak.
So when your heart decides to fail
let us not jump up and down on your chest
for you will never be the same again
do not confuse resuscitation with resurrection.

(Patient replies)
Doctor, I am dying
Pills and machines cannot save me now
Trials are merely hypothesis drafted in textbooks
giving false hope
to the ill.
So when God decides to call my name
do not bother jumping up and down on my chest
for I will be long gone by then
do not confuse body with soul.

Monica Pritchard, Year 4, as Cultural Competence

Be like you

Be like you
Talking like a 'southie'
Being more like you, please accept me
Trying to relate
Trying to be safe
Using words I've heard, street-talk I think
'Az' at the end of every word.

I hear my mouth say "gangsta" but I never say that
Slouching beside you
Cursing myself for dressing so proper
Wishing to look more like you
Trying to relate
Trying to be safe

Tilisi Puloka, Year 4, as Cultural Competence

A Thousand Words

Sitting in the consult room
staring blankly.
Me at you;
You at I.
Silence.

They told me you knew no English,
that communicating would be hard.
I didn't know your language;
I didn't know your culture.
How was I meant to play my part?

Time was ticking like a bomb.
Finally, I took a deep breath
looked you in the eye
with a broad, stiff, boat-shaped smile
"Where are you from?"

You smiled back, much more relaxed.
Then a conversation followed.
I wasn't sure what you understood.
Few worded questions, one worded answers,
smiles, shrugs and counting fingers.
Little in the way of speech
but a conversation nonetheless.

Some footsteps on the floor
a knock on the door
and the interpreter enters.
"Sorry I'm late, we can start now"

A picture paints a thousand words.
Pictures, we all understand.
A handshake with a big awkward smile
for us it had already been
a thousand words.

Alvan Cheng, Year 5, as Cultural Competence

Creative context

This poem describes an outpatient consultation with a Korean woman during which the interpreter was late. This experience reminded me that a large proportion of communication can be achieved non-verbally. In the doctor-patient relationship, the words we speak are important, but the meaning and feelings we communicate with basic rapport and simple body language can be easily forgotten.

Name

What would you have been
If the one you pray to
Had not an English reply

If your skin had not been
Piha beach sunset
If your hands had not
Thick Nikau palms
If your hair had not
Silver fern linings

Would I still know you
The way I do now?

Gerald Lee, Year 5, as Cultural Competence

Creative context
Inspired by my family who I often have language and cultural barriers with.

Shoulders and knees

The look on their faces, the outward disgust,
in this scantily clad woman, we wont put our trust.
See there, her shoulders! Are those really knees?
Never before have reactions like these
been what I faced when doing what I can
to take a history, do an exam.

In barely above the knee shorts
swallowing down any pissed off retorts
my shoulders you could hardly see,
(Need I add that it was thirty degrees)
to be discriminated against based on gender and dress
the reason behind which, I did quickly guess.

But of course, these actions I could not condone
regardless of how far away from my own
Religion values and cultural beliefs
could be, so I reflect and debrief.
For the first time it was me outside the norm
with patients taking little time to inform
reception that they'd absolutely not see
the medical student with her offensive knees.

This is the situation so many must face
when they feel apart because of language or race,
or religion or choices which others deem wrong.
When they are made to feel like they do not belong.
In a system where I quickly learned
it's a lot harder when the tables are turned.

Demi Poynter, Year 5, as Cultural Competence

Whaikorero

I stand alone
Before those gathered before me
"Kia ora e te whānau..."
My voice falters

I remember
Words
Kupu
Etched in memory
Orange ink on whiteboard
Repeating stanza
Repeating

Gathering myself
I carry on
"E te whare..."
I look heaven-wards
The rimu beams lie above me

"E te Kaupapa..."
I look around
I am surrounded
By friendly faces
Teachers, Kaumatua
Students, Tauira

"E Ngā Rangatira..."
The end is nearing
My words are strong
Filled with purpose
Meaning

Words of love
Words of hope
Words of light
Spoken words
Of a language that is nowhere near dying
I finish
Kua mutu.

James Enright, Year 4, as Cultural Competence

Creative context

Kura Po (night school) was a reprieve from the daily trials and tribulations of the clinical setting. During my general medicine rotation it maintained my sanity. The learning environment was relaxed and teachers worked alongside students to develop our understanding. In contrast, ward rounds were a constant source of stress and being lectured in front of others.

One week, I was the designated speaker for the students and I spoke a formal Whaikorero (speech) in the wharenui (meeting house). Prior to this I believed I lacked the confidence, the ability to complete this task. I thought that my voice would falter, fade out and die. I thought that my memory would fail me. I was wrong. I succeeded.

This experience shows that my cultural journey is a living process. It is more than words on paper. The Māori language is one of hope and new beginnings, not one of death. My time at Kura Po was a continuation of my journey to develop my understanding of Māori Dom, my culture, and my whakapapa (genealogy/history).

A forgotten promise

A promise to our forbears
A promise conveniently forgotten
Or a promise ignored?

This shouldn't be happening
Not now, not in our country
Not to those who deserve it least

Crowded houses
A feeding ground for illness
And for inequities to grow

That a sore throat could cause
So much hurt
Who could know?

History repeats itself

This is not a white man's disease
This is not equity
This is the remains of broken promises

We are the ambulance
At the bottom of the cliff
They deserve fences

Fight with bombs not bayonet
We were told
Five years ago now

Where are the bombs
When we need them
To repair this broken promise

Harry Alexander, Year 5, as Cultural Competence

Equal Justice

Call me EJ, do you know what that stands for?
Equal justice, yes equal justice
That is what I stand for.
It's been a big part of my career
What did I do you ask me? I was a musician
We sang songs with love, for love, for what we stood for
Not for money or fame, but for us
Equal justice, yes, for our people

I still sing songs for my grandchildren, they love me
When we all gather at the marae I sing songs
Matahuru Paparaangii is its name
Just out of Huntly
And they all gather and we eat the food our whānau makes
Yes we do
They are my big whanau and we love each other

You want to examine me? You sure can
I will let you touch my māhunga
Only because I like you and I know you understand this culture
But I don't let anyone just do that
A stranger cannot touch what is tapu
And draw the curtains please
And close the door
We don't want no aparangi in here

The wound looks bad? Yes it does
They say I need to have my katete, what's the word? Yes amputated
It's ok
The body is not as important as the spirit
It is just the vehicle. My mind will not change
And my spirit will also remain
My whanau will be here soon
Sorry dear you will not fit in this room with all them too
They'll come with the chaplain
And sing songs
And give me blessings
That will help me through

Ka kite an ō au I a koe kid
And never forget who you are
That is what makes you
Proud

Ruyan Chen, Year 4, as Cultural Competence

I am from

"So where are you from?"
And I pause

The pause grows; grows heavy with uncertainty.
What are they asking?

I scrutinise. I try bending the pause to yield meaning but it remains....
Such a simple question- it's no big deal- harmless-get over it- just tell them. Tell them what?

I am from my mother and from my father
From the life they forged, lived and left in Sri Lanka, all through sweat and sacrifice.
I am from a big family
From the more than a dozen siblings they had between them, who gave birth to my more than 20 cousins.
I am from my sister. She shares half my DNA and has shared every high and low of family life I have known
I am from multitudes like rain storms carving oceans into the earth

I am from Auckland
From what my parents built here. From every school I went to there; from every stitch in every uniform, every word written in an exam and every word heard from every teacher.
I am from every friend. The ones I no longer talk to and the ones I never want to stop talking to

From every glass of wine and every headache the morning after. From laughter and stress. From every school lunch my parents packed. From getting my eyebrows threaded. From failing my driving test. From coming out. From being a medical student.

I am from multitudes like trickling veins knitted into currents tumbling into a heart

I am from every wasted hour I spent wishing my skin to be whiter, my eyes lighter, my hair fairer and my name more pronounceable

"Oh I'm from Auckland
    "No but where are you (*really*) **from?**"
                    Not where you live- where you're from
        "Oh right **born** and bred?"
            "But what's your **background?**"

How did you come to be...why are you...here? When you look...

"Haha, um yeah, I was born in Sri Lanka and my parents moved here when I was four". The carcass of a smile stitched to my lips. My eyes yoked still lest they roll

The pause is filled with everything they wanted to know. It shrinks away from the multitudes taking with it a teardrop from the ocean
That's enough. I am from that drop. I am from what they know now and that's enough.
I am from elephants and spices and from humidity and sun I have only breathed for four years of my life and occasional holidays after
But that's enough and that's all

Shan Gunaratna, Year 5, as Cultural Competence

Health and Wellbeing

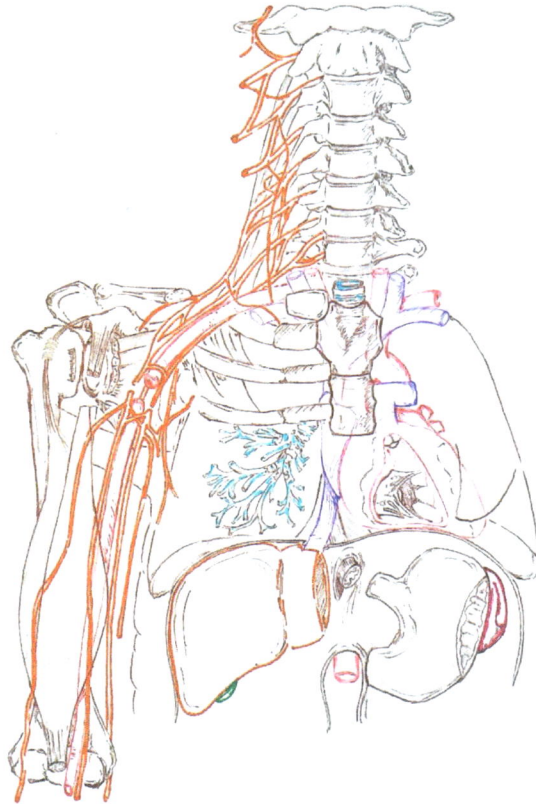

James Corbett, Year 4. *Coming together of clinical medicine.* 2016, (Back cover).

The Realities of Medical School

There once was a pre-med student called Jim,
who knew his chances of med school were slim,
When he got that email,
he had reason to hail
and nothing could erase his new-found grin.

There once was a second year called Tash.
She thought she would be happy at last.
She was keen and eager,
but found the rewards were meagre,
and realised her happiness had surpassed.

There once was a third year called Roger.
He was sick of lectures by old codgers,
so he skived off class,
scraped by on a pass,
and acquired the nickname of 'Dodger.'

There once was was a fourth year called Susannah.
She was always a meticulous planner,
but little did she know,
that when her hospital experience would grow
she would feel as if life had thrown her a spanner.

There once was a fifth year called Walter,
who felt like he never would falter.
When he failed his first OSCE,
he had no idea what 'came across me'.
At least his selective was in Malta.

There once was a TI called Joel.
He really engaged in his new role.
To finally have a purpose and to seem
like a legitimate part of his team
was incredibly soothing for the soul.

There once was a house officer called Kat,
who had never anticipated that,
she would be rushing around in a fray
charting medications all day,
Surely doctoring wasn't this crap?!

Anna Perera, Year 4, as Health & Wellbeing

Creative context
Medical school is a unique environment; a pressure cooker of sorts where one experiences a wide range of emotions. This poem is reflection, garnished with humour and mild cynicism, on some of my experiences and those of my colleagues.

Programming Error

I ripped the cartilage along the coast of your ribs
and opened your breath softly to me

Snuck down the rungs off your trachea into
the warm depths of a thousand tiny branches
making puckered microscopic homes
for tiny units all lined up.
Just single simple defenders against my invasion
and I could not break it.

I made a bed of the dome keeping apartheid
in your disintegrating body.
A musical whistle out, paper bag lungs crumpled;
and you sung me back out.

I remembered the feel of harsh
vibrations grating along my hands
unrelenting and despotic
leaving epithelial deposits along your bronchus
an intimate reminder of my exploration
long after you left the surgeon's interest.

But I forgot your name
ten minutes after I had learnt it.

T. J. Mitchell, Year 5, as Health & Wellbeing

Wild Frontiers

I am alone.
Engaged in these activities which
in some way
I find meaning.

I am a mortal engine.
A mere raft on the ocean
if not for the anchors of
love that tie me to
a shore that I call home.

I am here to learn art.
Yet, so easily how the capacity
to live ones art is chipped
away in a tender spur of carnage.

I am one pulse
on this beating Earth.
One thumb that sits abducted
by the pollicis brevis and
amongst this defiant frontier
it will not turn down.

Carmen Chan, Year 5, as Health & Wellbeing

Creative context

A song written in reminder to keep chasing the challenge, and to continually tackle the 'wild frontiers' of medicine. Written as I travelled into my fifth city for the year, for my medical attachments.

Acceptance

You won't remember me
fumbling with my hands
I shine a light into your eyes
and treat your body like my mother's collection of teacups

you don't remember the
odd questions that I asked
out of order, without structure
or pattern, somewhat medical

you wont remember me
you smile at me, like we've met before
we haven't of course
but it makes me smile too

you don't remember the
way my hands trembled
as I inserted a small needle
into your well mapped skin

you won't remember me
but you took my hand and told me
"you young thing, you are doing so well –
I am so proud of you"

you don't remember the
way your warm skin tempered mine
you won't remember me
and how a weight felt lifted off my shoulders

but I'll remember you

Holly Wilson, Year 4, as Health & Wellbeing

Dear Steve,

You do not know me.
And I do not know you.
But I am in your home, in your room.
And I am grateful to you
and your family
for letting me in - to be a part of your life
and your death.
The hospice nurse speaks in hushed tones introducing me
no one seems to mind, or even notice my presence.
I suppose you have had many people,
In
And out
Over the last two years.
Nurses and doctors, friends
and family
taking over your cares
as this disease has taken over your body.

Dear Steve,
You do not know me.
You look pained.
I am so sorry
I am so sorry that you have had to suffer like this.
Your daughter tells us in another room
that everyone is ready
everyone is prepared
that your suffering has endured far too long.
She is a strong girl
I do not know you, but I am sure you are so proud.

Dear Steve,
You do not know me.
And I do not know you.
But you are the same age as my father.
We are told, that not so long ago
you were so fit
so healthy
A marathon runner - a fast one too.
A strong supportive father
husband
friend.
Now, you can barely move
communicating with
your eyebrows and fingers
immobile
pained
silent
except for the rattle that resounds from your chest.
I am floored.

You are the same age as my father.

Dear Steve,
You do not know me
and I do not know you.
Goodbye, rest easy.
Thank – you

Hannah Gill, Year 5, as Health & Wellbeing

Spider

My bed is too large now
enough for me to curl up
enough for me to sprawl out
enough for me to stretch out my arm
and feel the cool sheets
draped over my skin.

My window is also too large now,
enough for me to gaze out at the clouds
and watch them roll by
like spectators drifting past an animal enclosure.

I am weak and I am small.
I am that spider
with a proud but empty web
coiling and recoiling with each gust of wind.

Months later, years later perhaps –
Who knows? Time is an owl
wise, attentive and purposeful.
– we may sit on a creaky bed again
with our legs like vines
twisted under dusty blankets.
Your nose cold
snuffling at the winter air
sharing a bowl of warm soup
and a bar of chocolate for dessert.

Even though you have gone
I still watch you sleep at night.
Your clumped mascara polluting my pillow
and your subtle wrinkles on your forehead
disappearing.
You sink into my soft chest
your body roughened by the trauma of heart break
as we begin to heal again.

Yushy Zhou, Year 4, as Health & Wellbeing

Poor Historian

Mr Taylor in room 5
can't remember
if he has diabetes, heart problems, or asthma.

We call him a *poor historian*
because his *history* is so *poor*
but really, that's on us, isn't it?

Listen again. Mr Taylor
is an *amazing* historian -
watch yesterday morning unfold.

He got up a bit late at six
last night was sweaty and hot
Funny for this time of year, right doc?

Ate five weetybix things with milk, lots of sugar
but then my tummy felt funny, did some big burps,
frightened the tuis squabbling in the kowhai tree.

Walked down to the river, with Jack, the old foxy,
like we've done every day
since Mary passed on, bless her.

Past the spot where I caught the biggest eel
wrangled up the glistening black coils
and everyone called it a monster.

Then over the rise I felt time catch me -
it's normal at seventy-four, right doc?
Couldn't catch my breath.

He is a marvelous historian.
On a bright, cool morning filled with bellbird chimes
and the rich brown stink of river mud
see the man with a stick clutch a fist to his chest
while his dog eyes the ducks in the water.

Sarah Shirley, Year 5, as Health & Wellbeing

Mouse

When we were finished
I refused to believe it.
I refused to accept it.
Even the stray blonde hair twined within the fabric of my woollen jumper
dry and brittle like a wisp of hard toffee
I kept.

The first few nights
I lay under the sheets that still lingered with your scent.
I breathed, deeply.
Trying desperately
to inhale what was left of your love
Our love.

Sometimes I would wake before daybreak
and sort through the memory boxes that were stored beneath my bed.
I would wipe the dust that had settled on them from the previous night
and pick through them
finding that I would lose a memory or two
each morning.

Perhaps the thief who was stealing our memories was a little mouse living in my
room
gnawing away at the old grainy photos
and dining on our messy handwritten notes to each other.
But not all thieves are wicked.
Each memory I lose of you is one less reason to smile
but also one less reason to sigh, to droop, and to cry.

The truth is
There is no mouse hiding under my bed
nibbling away at the memories we created.
I am the mouse
hungry for more time with you
a man deathly ill
digesting away at what little flesh remains
to stay alive.

The truth is,
Until I can riffle through the memory boxes beneath my bed
and be able to hold its jagged contents
without cutting my thin-skinned hands
I will leave the thousand odd boxes
one for each day I spent with you
undisturbed
so that the dust may settle again.

Yushy Zhou, Year 4, as Health & Wellbeing

Creative context

The poems are a part of series titled "Animals". They feature cameo appearances of household animals, and use direct metaphors relating to them in an attempt to describe my raw emotions and thoughts. These particular poems were written in the short days following the end of a three-year relationship.

Reflection on Anxiety

On days lacking inspiration, or a clarity of mind
I can find myself mistaking what is real and what is right
In a chaos that surrounds me, know I need a steady place
A light, a hope, a song, or even just a familiar face

It comes and goes in waves, never knowing where or when
The product of anxiety produced time and again
May catch me in the throat, or steal away my breath
I take solace in the knowledge that this isn't mental death

But knowledge takes a back seat when your heart is leaping out
And adrenaline takes over and you're overcome with doubt
Am I meant to be here? Do other people feel this way?
Why does there exist this constant battle in my brain?

Yet although a day seems cloudy, like respite may never come
A storm can't last forever, and so soon it shall be done
With roots that hold so firmly to a sanctity of thought
I shake away the negative emotions that I've caught

Though it may be a cycle, and these thoughts may reappear
They never can define me if I choose to conquer fear
If that which doesn't kill me makes me stronger, I must be
Heading on a path to find a better, stronger me.

Sophia Wilton, Year 4, as Health & Wellbeing

Creative context

Anxiety and depression are very common among medical students, as well as the general population. Despite this, I have found that it is something that is still considered quite taboo to talk about or discuss in a personal setting, yet I think it is something that needs to be acknowledged and accepted. I have written a poem that may show insight into a small aspect of my experience with anxiety and how it can affect day-to-day life.

Listen

This is Mr P.
He can't breathe.
Listen to his lungs.

This is Mr B.
He can't breathe.
Listen to his heart.

This is Mr G.
He is old.
Listen to his family.

This is Mrs K.
She is a woman.
Be careful, she has a uterus, and breasts.
Listen to her carefully, there is much to miss.

This is Miss L.
She feels tired and itchy.
Listen to her story of a waterfall in Thailand, mouth searing street food, and a night
with a German backpacker. Do not be jealous of travel, food, and sex.

This is Mr H.
He is Maori.
Be careful. Treat him *differently*, but do not *treat* him differently.
Listen to where he came from.

This is Mrs W.
She is dying.
Listen to the tick of the clock on the wall,
As you hold her small hand in yours.

Sarah Shirley, Year 5, as Health & Wellbeing

If You Want to Climb a Mountain, Begin at the Top

Staring down,
Vertical white slope
You idiot
It sure didn't look this high from the bottom

I'm slipping over the edge
The dreaded rush
The drop of the stomach
As I speed down
Eardrums popping
Vision blurring
Ski poles flaying
They aren't stopping me
Free falling into white
Nothing

I'm still at the top
Paralysed
Wait, was that all in my mind?
Let me be anywhere but here
Let my victories remain zero

But wait,
Who says I can't
What's the worst that can happen?
Beaten before I start, why, I'm cramping my own style

Clearing the hurdle
Is merely a task for the mind
To smash the steel barrier
Figuratively, of course
Is to beat my demons
Winning the battle against oneself
How to be a hero

Ski poles steady
Push myself forwards
Inch to the edge
Deep breathe –

Ruyan Chen, Year 4, as Health & Wellbeing

When the breathing mindfulness doesn't work

I remember sitting with her as she cried.
Her hands gripped mine
trembling.
Minutes earlier, she told me about the way her clothes looked like sheets
draped over a wiry frame
Only my ankles are fat, she said.
She smiles through tears when she remembers how she used to fly across
meadows, read books in trees.
In the GP clinic, she sits quietly
Now sleeping is enough exercise for me.
She came in with heart failure, but really she was here for the stress.
Each day I worry about dying, she said.
--- Stress strategies! I've learnt them!
But when I grapple my brain for mindfulness techniques, I realise that she cannot
do the breathing exercises
without feeling pain.
Yoga will not sooth her aching joints, her 4red bones.
So we sit and talk about trees and meadows,
of memories and stardust.
We sit in silence.
And then we pray.

Hannah Ng, 2016, Year 4, as Health & Wellbeing

Of Course

The surgeon in 302 thinks I'm a nurse,
he just called me Sister.
Excuse me mister, but I have a name.

That's what I wanted to say. But for shame
I did not.
For in this game
you nod, go fetch. You aim to
please - "Can you change her diaper?"
He said to me.

It's an adult incontinence product, Mr. Surgeon.
Not a diaper, nor a bib, not a cot or a crib,
But then she is not your mother.

She is 302.
Left Hip Arthroplasty under General Anaesthesia with Desflurane,
Nil by Mouth, No Known Allergies, Does not require return of body parts.

Oh good, one less bloody form to fill.

But my mouth fills and froths with the words I want to say to you.
Dark, sticky venom. It viciously clings to my throat
viscously tarry poison that hardens
like fear paving the roads ahead of me,
and then the words spill out like honey.

"Of course."

Always write angry letters to those who anger you, I was told.
Never mail them.
But this letter is not to you, Mr. Surgeon.
For you are simply a product, a conception
that since inception, has furthered the perception
That we are commanders; life givers and caretakers.
But patients should be patient, not movers and shakers.

No – this letter is to myself,
For I watch myself become and succumb
to the very thing I swore I wouldn't be.
"I want to help people" I told them in my medical interview.
[You can't change the world like this, you stupid girl.]

And yet
I will go fetch.
"I'm a medical student, by the way," I chortle.
It's not your fault, how could you know,
I should have corrected you earlier, sorry.
[Adjust your badge, tie your hair up tomorrow,
if you dressed better maybe people would take you seriously,
and stop talking. You're making a fool of yourself].

Above all tread carefully
for though his hands watchfully wield drills and diathermy,
he also holds your future, and he does not cradle that with care.

Go now and do.
Find the nurse for 302.
"Of course", I will say to you.

Natasha Trilokekar, Year 4, as Health & Wellbeing

Worth It? A poem about being a medical student

I stand there on ward round
With ten folders in my hand.
I scribble down what you say
As fast I can.
My hands are cramping,
There are sweat prints under my arms
And my feet are sogging wet.

I smile at each patient
And say 'good morning'.
I'm nodding and answering any
Questions you ask correctly.
I'm the perfect medical student,
You could have no concern about me.
I pay attention every moment of the day
And go the extra mile for nought credit.

Yet you don't know that I've just had
The third coffee of the morning,
That I spend my self-directed learning
Directing myself away from work.
You're unaware I was up till 5 this morning
Finishing a last minute assignment
Or that those tutorial I have every afternoon
Are spent drinking more coffee with my mates.

You probably don't care that
I ended my relationship last night
Or that I'm thousands of dollars in debt.
That I can't hear the murmur on the chest
Or see what is wrong on that ECG.

You don't know that I spend my days worrying
About not repeating the year,
About how I'm going to not end up as a GP,
About how I'm going to be able to buy my own house,
About how I'm not going to burnout
And most of all how I'm going to end up being like you.

But at the end of the day,
I'm happy with where I am.
What goes down, must come back up.
I look to the future
Where all the bad times pay off
And I can look back
And say
'It was all worth it'.....

Tom Doolin, Year 5, as Health & Wellbeing

Creative context

This poem captures some of the negative emotions that medical students can feel during clinical attachments and how you attempt to deal with these emotions.

Nameless

Do you know my name?

Do you know I have a family?

My husband looks worried, please reassure him

.......I'm ok

.......It's time

We knew this was coming

But did it have to happen like this...

Do you know my name?

You're all talking about me,

but not to me.

I can hear you,

I can feel you poking and tugging at me

My husband is watching, please be gentle

He can't see me like this

...because it's the last time

Do you even know my name?

Tilisi Puloka, Year 4, as Health & Wellbeing

Grief, Bereavement, Death and Loss

To me, grief, bereavement, death and loss
Is the image of how you looked that morning.
When I watched you take your final breath,
How you left this world without warning.

To me, grief, bereavement, death and loss
Is the fact that you won't ever see me grow.
I'm afraid you will not recognise me
I'm no longer the little girl you know.

To me, grief, bereavement, death and loss
Is knowing you won't be at my wedding.
To coach me through my first child's birth
every second of it, I'm dreading!

To me, grief, bereavement, death and loss
Is your absence on annual holidays.
I try to be grateful, I really do,
But I have no mama on Mother's Day.

To me, grief bereavement, death and loss
Is feeling abandoned, like I'm all alone.
People say I am now an orphan,
With no mama, no daddy and now no home.

To me, grief, bereavement, death and loss
Is knowing that I have to make do.
Though you've been gone for thirteen years now
Everyday my heart still cries for you.

To me, grief, bereavement, death and loss
Is why I have chosen this career.
While I know I can never bring you back,
I will help others when life is mean and unfair.

Aroha Ihaka, Year 5, as Health & Wellbeing

Creative context
I wrote this poem in my first year of medical school, reflecting on the death of my mother. Today, it gently reminds me of why I entered medical school and what it was like to be a family member of a terminally ill patient. It reminds me that my current patients are someone's mother, aunty, friend or sister and not simply someone with deranged LFT's or impressive clinical signs.

Two Days in E.D.

Worst Day

Grey jacket, grey hair, grey face,
he clutches his scarf to his chest
watching the rise and fall, rise and fall,
of the chest of the boy in the bed.

Two hours ago he found him,
a towing rope necklace around him,
suspended and dangling,
heartbroken and blue.

Best Day

There she goes, out the door,
her problem list trailing behind her:
diabetes (poorly controlled),
gout (painful),
chronic obstructive pulmonary disease (worsening),
osteoarthritis (crippling),
heart murmur (probably nothing),
paroxysmal atrial fibrillation (worrying).

She's back to her cats and her crosswords,
she'll be back here again in a month.

                        (I found the murmur)

                        Sarah Shirley, Year 5, as Health & Wellbeing

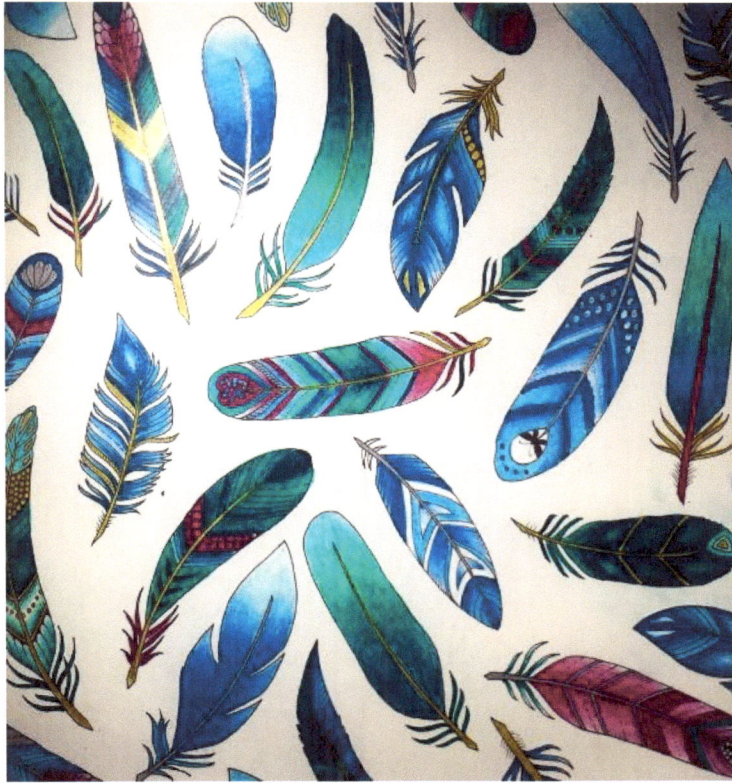

Demi Poynter, Year 5. *Meant to write reflection but I coloured instead*, 2016, as Health & Wellbeing.

Meant to write reflection but I coloured in instead

Meant to write a reflection but I coloured in instead,
A little bit of insight
to the workings of my head.

Thought I should include it,
Proof that I can see
That relaxing and not more work is the thing I need

How I ask, just one more task.
I never feel done
But the answer is absolutely not to deprive oneself of fun.

Try be a little mindful.
Quiet the endless chat
And a mere two hours later, your picture looks like that ⟸

Find a bit of balance
Don't be owned by stress
Only you yourself can protect your health, I will do no less.

Demi Poynter, Year 5 as Health & Wellbeing

The Face of Death

His face was one I had read about
An image from which textbook words had conjured
The face of one on St Peters doorstep
Ready to ring the doorbell

Skin stretched taut and white
A blank canvas
Coarse wrinkles scribbled haphazardly across
A painting void of colour

Each breath a ragged gasp
Of one running a marathon
Each pause just a fraction too long
I find myself gasping too

I shrug the hand of death from my shoulder
Like an unwanted garment
It falls to the floor and I leave it behind
Shivering in the new found cold

Aimee Humphries, Year 5, as Health & Wellbeing

Waiting for an invite.

When we are young we are jealous of the late nights, the bright lights, the television sights that we are not privy to
Then we grew as slaves to the long nights, up late at night, sleeping past the early lights and wasting time we feel entitled to
Growing older we are expected to rave into the night, drowning in the cellphone and laptop backlights, sleeping in classes we are not supposed to
Moving forward we study through the night, tell ourselves it is our right when striving for greater heights, that sleep comes second when we want to come first
Difficult to distinguish between day and night, nothing enthrals, enthuses or excites, willing yourself through your daily fight, knowing that this isn't even the worst
Chest tight
Midnight
Struggling to stay upright
Dreaming of one long, dark night that we are not invited to.

Teia Sebire, Year 4, as Health & Wellbeing

A Portrait by The Unrelenting Artist

Dedicated to the boy on the table

His face is frozen in youth
A snapshot of time lost
The haunting artwork of wasted prospects
Solemn work of one who does not rest

Eyes that should have seen a thousand more days
Blinking in the brightness of a new sun
Drinking in the smiles of a loved one
Forever closed to the darkest of nights

Hair swept off his face
Framing the last picture ever taken
Cut short and trim, never to grow again
Never to turn grey with age

Mouth parted just slightly
As if caught by surprise
The unexpected visit of The Artist unrelenting
A portrait we all pose for eventually

Aimee Humphries, Year 5, as Health & Wellbeing

Misc.

Don't fear
there are still a lot of things to learn

Like the shape of maps
and the reason for rings

where sunlight exists
and the way fish swim

what countries mean

the sounds of a moving camera in a homemade video
the sweetness of teeth
why life ends

how it begins

why it feels good for life to begin

why algae develop
and share codes
and make me

why clothes dry
and the sky looks flat

why cashews taste the same
and the decisions I make
don't

why are we all so different?

When information seems real
are our conclusions ever stronger than liquid?

be my detergent
play with my difference and
don't let me run out

Helen Ker, Year 5, as Health & Wellbeing

Little Shadow

Why do you follow me,
Little shadow?
Questioning everything I do.
Tugging at my pant legs
When I trail behind.
Carrying you makes me exhausted
And since you came into my life
I am so weary.
Tired right through me,
You sap my vitality from the inside,
Your sustenance.
Do others judge me when they see you?
Unwanted burden
I am trying to live with.
Brief escapist moments and
Fleeting pleasures
But you notice my inattention
Your low cry
I feel my reaction
 - My let down
And dread.
Will I never be free?
I guess it's my own fault anyway.

Take responsibility, persist,
And make lemonade
With this bitter fruit of life.

You can't adopt out depression.

Lizzi Wilson, Year 5, as Health & Wellbeing

Creative context
*This was written during my Obstetrics and Gynaecology attachment at Middlemore,
and learning about pst-natal depression, and reflecting on my own experiences of
depression.*

A Wayward World

Today I cried a little
For the man who lost his love
For the many who survive
For the child who did not eat

I cried for the woman
Who I passed along the way
With failing legs and metal frame
Who couldn't cross the street

More today than yesterday
I shed my solemn tears
For the old and decrepit souls
Whose loneliness I fear
I cast the drops and watch them fall
Each gently in the sand
To only see them swept away
Like tides that claim the land

And so each day I cry a little
For the world has lost its way
For losing hope in others
For feeling, this way – each day

If only tears of sadness
Gave all the power to change
To see beyond the madness
That comes from judging skin

But throughout time and time again
We galvanize the hurt
Prey upon each other
Until ruin comes or worse

So today I say ye cry a little
For the lost and wayward world
And fear thee not that we're alone
In this you have to know.

Coll Campbell, Year 4, as Health & Wellbeing

Creative context

As doctors and as human beings we all share unique similarities with one another. One similarity is that our consciousness allows us to all have a uniquely individual experience. For some, this can be a somewhat lonely and melancholic experience if we feel judged by others for any number of reasons. Age, sex, attractiveness, income, skin-colour, religious faith, size, no matter who we interact with, none of it should matter. It shouldn't matter because knowing we all share the same existential code that drives both our deepest happiness and fears, ultimately connects us. Having this awareness, there is then a duty to raise people up because we empathise with the vicissitudes of the human condition.

Base Pairs

Some nights you feel rough around the edges - or maybe it's that you become hyperaware of your rough edges, edges that might tear skin if you ran your fingers across them in the wrong way.
You become aware of your mortality.
You're just bone and blood and arteries all caught up somehow inside skin that bruises and scars.
It's easy to forget.
But it's also an easy thing to get tangled in, until it's the only thing in your head.
You want to run a very hot bath and
sit in the water chipping away
at your nail polish until it's all gone,
until your nails are bare,
until the water's turned your skin so
soft and wrinkled you think it could fall
right off.
A pairs with T.
C pairs with G.
And that's all we'll ever be.

Alice Hunter, Year 4, as Health & Wellbeing

Call me change

We are born,
Pluripotent stem cells,
With all the potential
To be anything in the world!
A nerve cell, a muscle fibre, a hepatocyte.

We differentiate along these pathways,
According to our environments;
The signals and the cells around us.
We become more functional and specialised,
Fit into a tight niche in this world.

But, as we differentiate,
We forget,
How to be anything else
We could have been;
We lose touch with our sister stem cells,
Who are now surfactant, endothelial and osteoblast cells.

We make structures with divisions, walls,
Categorise by type and exteriorly displayed antigens,
Kept discrete by our labels.
Guard cells patrol
For anyone 'different'.

We perform set tasks
Live set lives,
Die at set times.

But I remember.
I remember what it is to be free
To choose my own destiny,
To make my own way in life
- And to grow.

I am changing.
Losing my function, my attachment to this –
My assigned place in the mud.
I will not be another brick in your wall;
Another cog in your factory.

I will expand and move,
Beyond the future destined
By this system's double helix tracks;

I will re-join my sisters and reconnect;
They will remember what it is to be anything
Be free like me.

They will try to resist me
Chop me down
Take me out
And poison me;
But if there are enough of us, we can overcome them,
Disrupt this system
For a new future.

Call me change.

Lizzi Wilson, Year 5, as Health & Wellbeing

Creative context
This is a piece written about the way our hospital and the health system takes us and shapes us into departments and titles and names, and then we learn to perform specialized tasks and functions much like differentiating cells, and I used the image of cancer to illustrate change.

Time to Rest

Rushing on the highway like a boy racer
Just a little too late to
Hear her last breath

She lay
Eyes closed and hands still gently warm
Her yellow skin so foreign to my faltering gaze

I squeezed my sister's hand tight
Sharing the knowledge, that no more would we hear her sharp staccato rhythm
Scolding us for not eating her food

Yet no tears fell
As useless as an ornament I stood
Was it grief, or relief, I felt the strongest?

Too many long nights
Too many aches
Too many hopes
Disintegrated

Days later, in line we stood
Watching the wooden box slide into red flames
Finality

Only then did it hit
The strike of the gong mimicking the snap
Of the heartstring
Finally the gates opened to let the flood through

We prayed through the night
To ease our minds, the
Emptiness, filled by each other's presence

As I looked across the haze rising from the incense
At my mum, face drawn and back bent
I felt infinitely comforted by her presence

Life goes on
And ever more the reason to appreciate
What is in front of us now.

Ruyan Chen, Year 4, as Health & Wellbeing

Fitzroy

My heart aches for places
And wilderness spaces
I know like the back of my hand.

Skies stretch, infinite
And faces smile, intimate
And wine always in demand!

Campfires are built
Amongst the red silt
As time slows under these stars.

Lit up by the moon
The sight makes me swoon
Swags and 4 x 4 cars.

"Sister", not student
and laughs are abundant
we learn to be more than we are

Where the patients are teachers
And doctors are preachers
I learn medicine is really an art.

Connections are made,
A toy guitar played,
I put down my roots deep.

Sunsets and friends
Beginnings and ends
Leaving is making me weep…

Red tracks still to explore
My heart yearns for more
And people I still haven't met

Oh, I will come back
You can be sure of that
I'm not done with the Kimberley yet!

For the beauty and laughs
And good times with the staff
Fitzroy, au revoir.

Lizzi Wilson, Year 5, as Health & Wellbeing

Creative context
I wrote this about my Selective placement in a tiny Aboriginal town in remote Western Australia called Fitzroy Crossing with the most incredible people. I learnt more from the patients, who called the local girls "sister," than from the locum doctors. I spent most weekends around a campfire playing guitar under a sky full of stars, with the nurses and workers not on shift. I absolutely loved "Fitty"!

Doctor for a doctor

I can help you
No cause for concern
Let me reassure you
Cure we'll discern

Doctor to patient
The adage goes
I will be here for you
You already know.

Bones aching
Mind racing
A million things waiting
Unforgiving parking
Attention waning
Paining
Crying
Breaking

Who is the patient?
Who needs who?

Who helps the help-
If it's you who needs you?

The adage is incomplete-
The massage chain cheats
Where does the doctor go-
Do you see what I mean?

Doctor to doctor
We need to know
That reassurance is not limited
To telling someone else so

Doctor to doctor
It should also go

Because aching bones
Can't bear the weight of stethoscope.

-Manasi Deshpande, Year 5, as Health & Wellbeing

Creative context
In order to honour the deep privilege we have to serve others in this profession; it is essential to prioritise our own health and wellbeing. Doing so ensures we are the best versions of ourselves for those whom we are caring for.

A Clear Head and a Dark Heart

Two neurological emergencies
One man, aged 47
One woman, aged 74
One put to sleep, not knowing he will never wake up
One waking up, not knowing how close she came to death

Crowds and chaos surround the CT scan
Brightness. Haemorrhage. The crowds retreat
Darkness. Ischemia. The crowds advance
All is now clear, in black and white, to everyone but me
One we can attempt to save, and one to just let be

Deflated by hopeless limitation
Uplifted by cutting-edge sophistication
These tools of our trade: the pill and the knife
I look on as a brain slowly bleeds to death
and as blood flow restores a brain to life

Action not taken, for too much to lose
Action undertaken, for nothing to lose
At the end of the day, did the scan really choose?
It's not just the heaviness of their own heads
that is carried on those shoulders

Two patients – same signs, different outcomes
One heart returned a flatline
One brain returned to baseline
The symmetry in their differences
Help bring some comfort to me

-Ursula Byrne, Year 5, as Health & Wellbeing

Resilience

Through time a tale transcends,
Words immortalized,
A love locked and caged and lost within its own universe.

I call out to you, but you do not
Hear, the echoes of my voice
Floating –
A chasm separates us.

There is a new light for both of us,
One we desperately grasp for.
But as we leave each other behind
Let our love dance, swirl,
Swirl
Amongst stolen glances and silenced cries.

Warped memories and the
Clarity
Of two hearts once wrapped in one.

My strength, my pain, it's in my eyes
And it's giving me away.
And you, your strength, your pain
Will live beyond.

You are now my moon
And as you glow, I am warm.

Thoughts on losing the one you love

A good day,
A bad day.

A bad day,
A worse day.

A worse week,
A good minute.

A minute is all I need.

For I am stronger than my own emotions,
And carrying someone else,
Holding their trust in my hands,
Holding their heart in my heart,
Is all I need
Even for a minute
To get back up again.

Hold another's life

As if it were as fragile as glass.
We are all breakable.
And being there for someone makes it all worth it.

Reasons to keep going

Aishwarya Joshi, Year 4, as Health & Wellbeing

Creative context
Medicine privileges us with the ability to hold patient's hopes and fears in the most intimate of ways. We are tasked with treating individuals, and sometimes, we are tasked with facing the grief of their loved ones. This piece of writing reflects acceptance of grief, serving as a reminder that it is through compassion for our patients that we are able to stay resilient alongside them.

She's gone

Sitting, sleeping, drooling on my hand.
I'm shattered awake by the insistent beep,
the shrill nag of a heart ceased.
They come and brush me out
- as if I wasn't wanting to go anyway
Seconds later, muffled thud of an electro-live body.
Then the sadden hesitance of my name,
betrays what they will say.
'Nothing we could do sorry, she had already gone'
For once they couldn't be more right.
But their timing is wrong, it wasn't just now.
Ever since she peed in the shower
or stored milk in the oven, she'd gone.
Dylan, she'd said, my mind is wandering away
My name's Matt, Mum; and don't worry it'll come back.
And it did, after a time - long or short, till that evening.
That evening it didn't, it must have got lost,
or has fallen over, I guess we will never know.
It just took her body a while to give up,
lose that hope of a tearful reunion.

Allie Rout, 2015, Year 3*

*In response to an invitation to have *Breaking* included in this collection Allie
agreed and also put forward this second poem, *She's Gone*, which could be
considered as Health & Wellbeing.

I Hope to Be a Doctor

I hope to be a doctor in the morning

Who will answer patients' woes and worries

Who will make time despite the panic and stress

Who will not be afraid to ask seniors for help when required

I hope to be a doctor in the afternoon

Who will not let time control my actions and thoughts

Who will finish tasks promptly and in an appropriate manner

Who will do my job whole heartedly with a smile beaming on my face

I hope to be a doctor in the evening

Who will support my collegues and peers overnight and hope for the same

Who will find a balance between work and home life

Who will cook, clean and look after my family with the same care I give my patients

I hope to be a doctor everyday

Who will never betray a friend to advance my career path

Who will acknowledge there are things out of my control

Who will think in the present and not be stuck in the past

Anonymous, as Health & Wellbeing

Following me home

Orthopaedic round.
"he's avulsed the cartilage of his Talus, needs a fusion"
We trail in like ants
I pull the soundproof curtain
"do you understand the surgery?"
"They said something about a fusion.
 will I still be able to move the ankle?"
"No"
"you'll get about 20 degrees from the mid tarsal joint"
"Can I run?"
"No"
"walk?"
"It'll be harder"
He's 19 years old

"How was your day?"
"It was cool, I got to pull out a K-wire"

Lying down
The day swirls around my head
I looked at his face.
Eyes cast down
His face found its shadow
Can't sleep

Pain round.
"He's got acute pancreatitis"
"drinks a bottle of wine a day"
"His dad died of the same thing"
"How are you feeling?"
"Not very good, the nurses wouldn't let me have any of the good stuff for
saint paddys"
Still sore
More morphine

"How was your day?"
"it was good, finished early"

Sitting down.
Mind wanders, finds the memory
My thorax explodes
Fits of laughter
Black humor
The cruel vice of a hardening heart

Colorectal clinic.
"Next one has cancer of the rectum"
"do you mind if the medical student sits in?"

"No it's fine"
"Any other medical problems?"
"My father raped me when I was a little girl"
"The doctors said I should mention it for anything down there"
"In case that's what caused it"

"How was your day?"
"It was hard"
"Want to talk about it?"
"Yes"

"Clap, Clap Clap"
My shoes flick up the sand
The sun casts its amber gaze over the Mount
Dogs run along the beach and children play in the surf.
Hospital seems far away
The world shifts back into perspective

Eddie Hughes, Year 4, as Health & Wellbeing

Creative context
I wrote this poem (Following me home) about struggling to adapt to the clinical environment and having to see and hear a lot of sad and unpleasant things. Entering the clinical environment has made me realise I had internalised a lot of "old world" medical views about dealing with upsetting experiences like compartmentalising clinical and home life or using gallows humour. Rejecting these ideas and learning to accept help and talk about experiences, rather than bottling them up, has been very important for me in learning to be resilient in the clinical environment.

Leaving Good for Great
(12ᵗʰ March 2016)

I feel like I'm constantly trying,

To tread on, and balance the line,

Between ordinary,

And going for something extra.

Everyone is plugged into this world at a base level,

And I know I need to maintain this connection.

But I want to extend myself beyond it,

Extend onto the upper levels.

One part filled with the excitement of stepping forward,

Into the future, into the unknown.

But two parts cling to the fear of leaving everything,

Everything that's comfy and all that is known.

But this balancing act, while it may seem 'fine',

Its very existence creates strain.

It feels like I'm splitting,

Torn between worlds.

Between safety and success.

These two groups of people who inspire, support and connect,

Bringing me more joy than I could ever think was possible.

And alone in the middle is me.

Not stepping in, not stepping out.

This hokey-pokey of isolation.

A fine line in a mist of uncertainty,

Constant second guessing,

And roller-coaster rides of inspiration, motivation and persistence on the uphills,

Followed by doubt, insecurity and fear pervading the downhills.

This daily grind seems long and arduous,

With only a faint light at the end of the tunnel:

The very goals I hold so high and lofty.

This creates the determination to continue,

To continue on with this balancing act.

I try to tell myself,

"Do not be afraid,

Of leaving good, for great".

But is this tug of war, really a way to live?

Nikhil Magan, Year 5, as Health & Wellbeing

Creative context

This poem aims to highlight the – often subconscious – inner conflict between your willingness to take the 'easy road' and be happy, relax and enjoy right now, in contrast to the 'hard road' which requires sacrifice, hard work, motivation and persistence. In particular, it identifies with those who reside in the middle, whose journeys seem to take them somewhere in between without really fulfilling either path.

Gazelle

Strip off warmth and comfort,
Pull on singlet and shorts.
The sky is moody, spits and threatens,
But a little water does not frighten me.

Slip into worn shoes,
Laces so well stretched by the kilometres.
My feet enter vessels that embrace the irregularities
Of these funny looking things, four friends reuniting.

Slam the door, turn the key,
Plug me into a world of sound.
The familiar chords chime,
My heart leaps, anticipating.

Beginning workout.

Freed from a cage. Set loose:
Just me, the music and my own two feet.
Off flying, ascending to the peaks,
I am invincible.

Breathing becomes heavy,
Heartbeats thunder in my ears.
I punish the earth under my tread;
I hold my head high. I do not stop.

I would know these footpaths blinded,
Every hill a familiar adversary.
Gentle slopes calm gasps to sighs, and soon,
Respite – the road that leads me home.

High and giddy, I have conquered,
The edges of the world are sharp, impossibly defined.
With slowing breaths, clarity descends:
This is what it means to be alive.

Euphemia Li, Year 4, as Health & Wellbeing

Here Not There

Darkness, light
The eternal fight
Here or there
Which one, when

Confused identity
Never settling
Here or there
Which one, when

I choose light
My choice is slight

Commitment seems strong
Not for long

Anger, frustration, sadness, pain
Will to go on, starting to wain

Alone, again
Alone, again
Alone, again
Alone, again

Alone is a choice
Make it or not
Here or there
Which one, when

I choose light
I'm not alone
I am here not there
For now

Mark Walus, Year 4, as Health & Wellbeing

Learning & Teaching

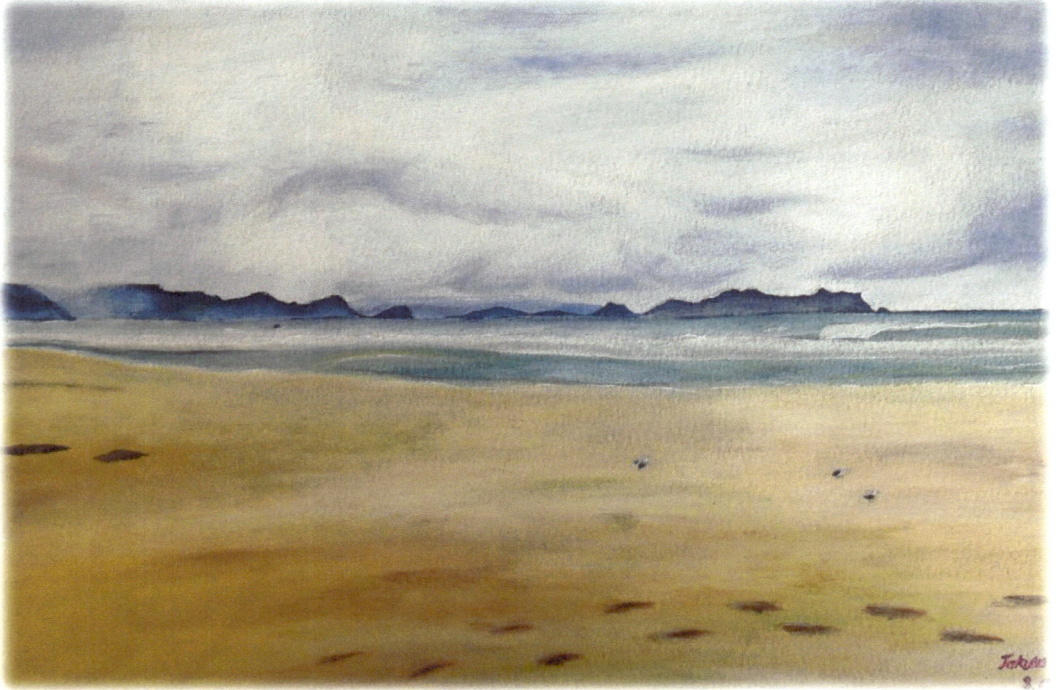

Joanna Davie, Year 5. *Takou Bay, Northland*. April 2016.

Half past three

They come in with pale, blotched faces,
Trying not to worry
About what comes next

My wife is pregnant - he says
Yes, we've had a scan
Just last week in fact
The baby was fine
Brady-cardiac though

This morning my wife started bleeding
Along with abdominal pain
We are from New York
I am a physician

We know this could be nothing,
But it could be something,
We would just like to know, Sir

They thanked me on the way out
Shook my hand
Wished me luck with my studies

It was something

Holly Wilson, Year 4, as Learning & Teaching

The Obs and Gynae* Feedback Session

Was it really feedback?

I had prepared well.
I had studied and practiced, then studied and practiced.
I turned up on the day feeling nervous, but at ease.
I had prepared well.

We completed the OSCE.
It was a tumultuous experience.
They changed the format completely.
We were told to focus on management and yet everywhere was 'take a history'.
I felt as though I had failed both my clinical team and myself.
We completed the OSCE.

Her station was about Gestational Diabetes.
She held her marking schedule up so we couldn't make eye contact.
She answered yes or no, so rapport couldn't be established.
She questioned students on whether they had even read the vignette.
She spoke bluntly; ruder than any patient I had ever seen.
Her station was about Gestational Diabetes.

They held a feedback session at the end.
We shared a defeated look as we discussed.
They asked us what could be improved, we told them.
She debated us at every point.
How can the same comments from every participant be wrong?
They held a feedback session at the end.

I felt defeated.
I had prepared myself for the assessment.
I did not know that the format would change.
We worked hard and now questioned our own ability to pass.
I felt defeated.

Anonymous, as Learning & Teaching

*Obstetrics & Gynaecology

The Surgeon

He stands towering over the group.
Immaculately dressed,
in a freshly pressed shirt,
sleeves rolled up
with surgical precision.

His every action
was met with a flurry of movement.
A person furiously scribed
Him word for word,
while another darted down a corridor
into oblivion.

His clenched fist
Rapped on the patient's door.
'Good morning'
He gently mumbled,
smiling through old,
wise eyes.

He perched Himself precariously
at the edge of the bed.
He examined her abdomen,
gently palpating it.
she giggled pearls of laughter
in response.

Not all surgeons
bite.

Connor Kim, Year 5, as Learning & Teaching

Unwanted knowledge

The unwanted knowledge, passed high to low.

Things more damaging than warranted

a slipped misspoken word

the shying away from touch

the brusque brutality of the uncaring

hands harbouring harm, uncleaned

short, snappish demands.

Those things we try not emulate

But

eventually capitulate

becoming as those we strove not to.

Xavier Field, Year 4, as Learning & Teaching

The *hidden* hidden curriculum

-A cynically honest summary of the first clinical year.

Day one in the hospital
our nerves as high as our hope.
What is our role in the hospital?
It's however long is a piece of rope.

We start with faith in the scheme
and faith in what we've been taught.
Finally entering the hospital is like a dream
But nothing is anything like what we thought.

We're told pull the curtains shut well
to have a meaningful role in your team.
And hold the patient's notes tightly
never mind about your self-esteem.

"The grumpy man who had a stroke with a walking stick,"
"The old lady with a chest infection."
Avoiding emotional attachment to the sick
is done by maximising disconnection.

Talk with your back to the patient
and with words which they're sure to not understand.
This will ensure they'll want to leave with a sprint
but your team still thinks your grand.

Blood, cancer and death used to be such a big deal
but expressing your surprise at this is despised.
The biggest change you undergo during the year
is certainly becoming desensitised.

You work hard for a full six weeks
it all comes down to some boxes being ticked.
You'll get a pass no matter your techniques
it's a curse if you're trying to be perfect.

Travel to and from the hospital on your own
feeling alone despite surrounded by many others.
My only real support is 950 kilometres away
and this is my mother's.

Simply because I'm a female
every day I'm asked if I'm training to be a nurse.
When I thought sexism was only tale
I hope being this gender doesn't become a curse.

Should I be myself today?
or simply fit into someone else's mould.
What is the right thing to say?
We are never really told.

Clinical years aren't all this bad
although balancing all your priorities can be a handful.
There is still a lot of fun to be had
and many days are extremely gainful.

Although as a student we often have little influence
if in the nine months we are on the ward
we are able to make a difference to just one patient
to me that is enough of a reward.

Megan de Lambert, Year 4, as Learning & Teaching

Organic cotton hats

"They are happy to have you in the room" said the nurse
And so with bumbling feet and scratchy scrubs
I shuffled across the room
Excited to witness my first caesarean section

The expecting parents were waiting inside
Mike owned his own company
Jenny ran a childcare business
The soon to be Charlotte would be their third child

Preparation and security hung in the air
As tangible as the drapes from which Charlotte would soon emerge
A hat and blanket lay waiting expectantly
All organic cotton (of course)

And one hour later, the excitement was over
Mum and baby wheeled away for rest
Grandparents called, siblings introduced
Charlotte slotting easily into her new life

"They are happy to have you in the room" said the nurse
And so half an hour later, with bumbling feet and scratchy scrubs
I shuffled across the room
Excited to witness my second caesarean section

The expecting parents were waiting inside
Tane was a truck driver, just made redundant
Mania was on the unemployment benefit
The soon to be Tamati was their first child

Anxiety and apprehension pasted itself
Over the young parent's faces
Conversations not about what the baby would look like
But how they would get home with a broken down car

And when Tamati was brought into this world
There was nothing remotely organic
About the synthetic hospital hat placed on his head
Nor the mixed reaction his presence brought

On that day, two emergency caesarean sections happened
Same theatre, same staff, same operating bed
Two little lives brought into the world
Both perfectly formed, and beautiful

Yet from the second the bed left the theatre
Those two little lives' journeys parted ways forever
Their similarities ceasing as indiscreetly

As the fabric making up their different hats

And meanwhile tucked away in the corner
Stood myself, a small student
Insignificant to most
Yet undoubtedly witnessing the lottery of life

Emily Aitken, Year 5, as Learning & Teaching

Creative context
During my Obstetrics run, I had the privilege of observing two emergency caesarean sections one after the other and subsequently found myself witnessing first-hand how from the moment a child is born, certain environmental conditions and inequalities set a baby's life tangent into motion. Despite being born in similar circumstances, it was evident that these two babies would lead extremely different lives.

You've Taught Me

You've taught me to medicate their pain and strife,
You've taught me that workplace stress is a way of life.
You've taught me how to take a blood gas,
You've taught me to discharge patients fast.
You've taught me the parameters of chronic renal failure,
You've taught me to roll your eyes when we speak to her.
You've taught me vertigo presentations and how to solve them,
You've taught me not to act if it's not your problem.
You've taught me the properties of lignocaine,
You've taught me my place in the food chain.
You've taught me to call patients by their name,
You've taught me that you're never to blame.
But if there's one thing that I have come to know,
You've taught me that even the best doctors have room to grow.

Marija Zutic, Year 4, as Learning & Teaching

Paediatric Experiences

Homelessness
Coldness
Chronic and terminal illnesses
Helplessness
Breathless
Clonus and meningitides
Carelessness
Sadness
Paediatric experiences

Hannah Smiley, Year 5, as Learning & Teaching

Medical School Learning

A desk drawer ajar with notes
A coffee mugs prurient smell of age
The late nights under coarse light
With blisters defining repetitive pen strokes
A ritual defined by ink on paper
By used coffee cups and bags under my eyes

The gentle yearning for more knowledge
The learned lists, the diagrams, anatomy, pathology, physiology
The ritual ward rounds - signs galore
The learning at home, in labs, the hospital
I must learn enough, enough to survive house officer

Hippocrates to Osler and all between
Clinical methods to advance ones skills
Bedside teaching, murmurs and heaves
All knowledge is free, but what is free in return we must pay
With time to give back, to those who need our aid

And so at my desk, it is late and I'm tired
Another page of notes confirmed to my brain for tomorrow
To reflect back on a year, where I have for the first time
Experienced how that learning is applied,
To the real life situation the patient in hospital
From learnt knowledge in a book, to learnt knowledge on a stethoscope

I can see the road ahead is long
The medical encyclopedia is extensive, the patients more complex than ever
But my learning will not cease and my skill only increase
Until it is my turn to pass on the knowledge to those below me

So in one year I will reflect on the end of medical school, the highs, the lows, the
knowledge, the sacrifice
And I will begin a new chapter like all those before
And I know there will be more to learn
And I know I will always have something to give, something to teach
Whether it is my friend, my family, my patient, my colleague, my people

Anonymous, as Learning & Teaching

A Good Teacher

In Medical School,
We learn many things that are cool
However, some things are difficult
making me feel a fool
If the teacher is a jewel
I will not be in a whirlpool

If a teacher is good,
there will be no rude-
awakening
What is a good teacher one may ask?

A Good Teacher Is One that Never Preaches,
But instead exemplifies
such that the Knowledge amplifies the practice
From suturing to nurturing,
patience is a must

In a pool of blood around a patient's thumb
I was asked to suture such that his
thumb had a future
Who would have known?

When teaching injecting to reflecting
a teacher that is not only correcting but also inspecting
will have the students respecting

In medical school,
the content we learn is often cool
from the anatomy of veins to the
characteristics of pain.

Over the year, I have prepared
for my career.
Many an hour has been spent turning
pages earning my learning

With a good teacher however,
I am made to feel more clever.
and my learning is better.

Kathryn McMonagle, Year 5, as Learning & Teaching

Building your skills

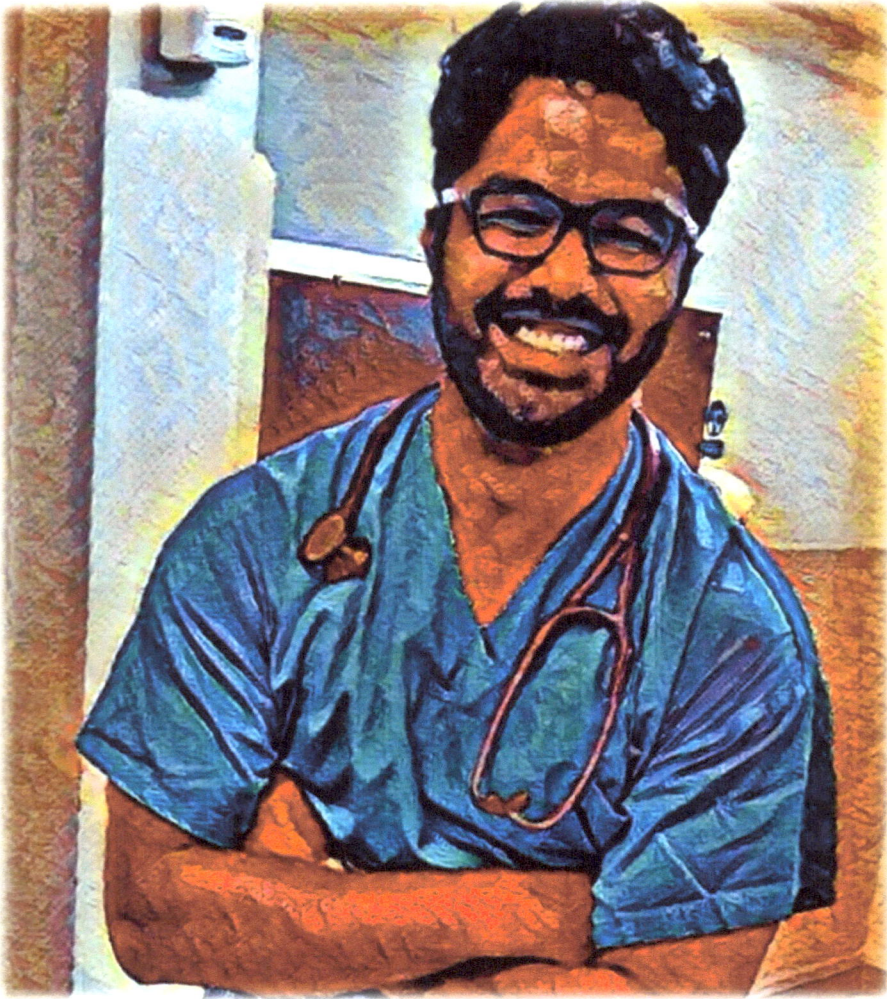

Coll Campbell, Year 4. *Self-portrait*. 2016.

Creative context

Here I am chuffed with my scrubs on the first day of 4th Year Medicine and the first day of General Surgery.

Creativity as self-care and a clinical skill

Sharyn Esteves

It's easy to think we are not creative. That creativity is synonymous with needing to have 'talent' or innate artistic ability. I certainly spent many years thinking I was not a creative person. Bland marks in art at high school, a sense that I had no ability and an affinity for the scientific meant the subject was dropped at the first opportunity for a focus on the sciences. Often, an expressed desire to study medicine means being purposively funnelled into the sciences and away from the arts and social sciences, as if somehow they are mutually exclusive.

Working as a doctor certainly brings its stressful moments and burnout remains problematic for the profession (23). Over the last few decades there has been a recognition that self care of the individual is an important part of managing such work related stress. (24). Such that self care is now recognised as part of medical professionalism, the idea being well-rounded individuals – with creative interests, and who attend to aspects of their lives outside medicine – are better able manage the stresses that their jobs bring. But as well as a means of caring for self, there is also a different focus emerging in the literature; that creativity is, in fact, fundamental to the practice of medicine – an actual clinical skill. (25)

There is an evolving movement to include more creativity in medical undergraduate curricula. This has mostly taken the form of the inclusion of humanities courses, to help students understand the social, cultural, creative and artistic sides of medicine; rather than focusing purely on the technical side. Engaging with the humanities is seen as a way for students to explore and make sense of their experiences in the clinical learning environment, to help them better understand patients' experiences with an aim of improving compassion and empathy. One medical school has gone as far as making creativity a compulsory component of the curriculum, where students are required to submit creative pieces of work for assessment.(26)

In a recent paper 'Doctors as Makers,' Baruch (25) proposes that creative thinking promotes dealing with the complexity and ambiguity found in everyday medical practice and discusses the concept of creative skills as valuable clinical skills. He argues that one of the roles of a doctor should be 'maker' – a creative artistic role. Developing medical students' skills to question, explore and challenge clinical encounters allows them to develop a certain comfort with 'not knowing,' helping them confront the intricacy and complications oft found in modern medicine. Baruch concludes that "By taking students out of their comfort zones and encouraging them to think critically and creatively about medical practice, maybe we will provide a generative space for them to understand their place in it..... Maybe they will ask different types of questions, engage in conversations, seek compassionate solutions – not because they are striving to be more empathic, but rather, because they are trying to be more creative" (2017: 43).

Personally, the emergence of creativity has been a gradual awakening. It began with a small internal voice questioning, what it would be like to be able draw and paint? A night class here and a few weekend courses there finally culminated in a Diploma of Art and Design. With the realisation that I can be both a doctor and an artist, the positive effects on both my private and work life cannot be overstated. As a confirmation of the points discussed above, it has been both a means of active self-care, as well as realising that the actual process of making art – the curiosity and exploration with the constant interpretation to make meaning – has actively fed into my clinical practice to deliver holistic patient centred care in my current work as a Palliative Care doctor. And for that I will be forever grateful.

So it's very encouraging to see medical students demonstrating their creativity in their reflective portfolios, including pieces of work that are trying to make meaning of complex interactions within the clinical learning environment. We hope that this collection of work from Year Four and Year Five medical students' portfolios will showcase the creativity that is occurring within our medical programme and encourage more students to focus on developing this important skill.

"Physicians must identify, nurture, and defend their personal interests and values if they desire personal and professional satisfaction in life." (24)

"Creativity is not a luxury, it is an essential component of the innovation on which the future of our health service depends." (26)

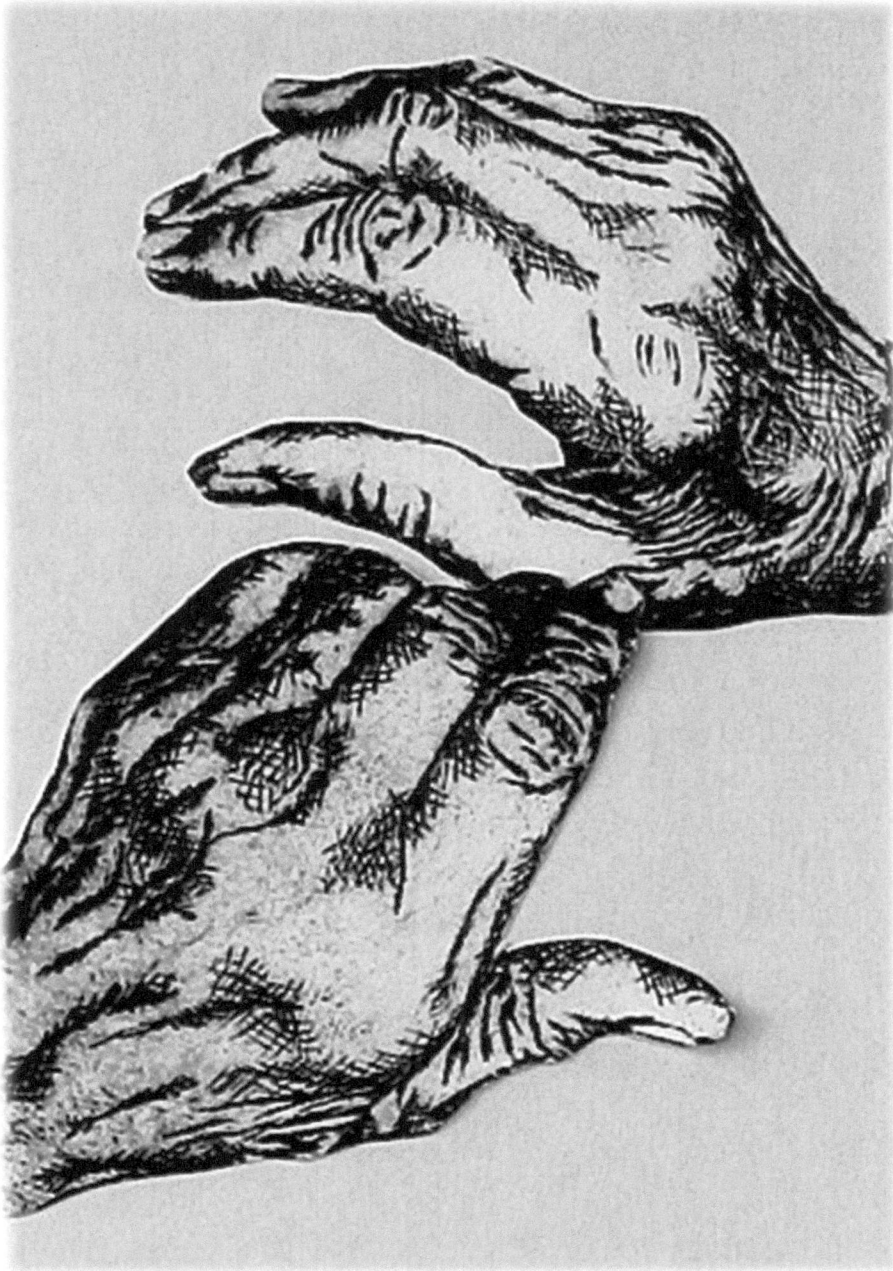

Helen Kandelaki, Year 4. *Bereavement*. 2016.

Three steps toward poetry

Lisa Samuels

Welcoming thoughts

Poetry gives language a chance to dream itself. It lets writers and readers get closer to our most important meaning-making tool – language – in a discovery-oriented, door-opening environment. Opening the doors of our language cultivates mental freedom for us.

Written for the relative newcomer, this essay adumbrates three steps to writing poetry: Prepare, Compose, and Revise. Ideally, each step happens separately so it can happen fully. These are practice-based steps: not about sudden realization of knowledge content, but about creating the conditions for inspiration. Some brief examples are provided, but there's much more to talk about.

1. Prepare

There is no such thing as a blank page. Language is already on the move in you, in the world, and in the page and screen: we can think of this as the bio-history and intertextuality of language. To make a poem opportunity happen, it is helpful to choose an approach to writing a new poem and then arrange the materials and context you need for that approach.

What is sometimes called "free writing" – writing whatever you want in whatever manner for however long – tends to call upon our default language patterns. These are the patterns we want to expand and strengthen, so that there are more language patterns in our repertoire.

"Proceduralism" works from the other end: this term describes **poetry whose formal characteristics are mostly determined in advance of composition. Sonnets, sestinas, or "formal imitation" (using the exact same shapes as a poem that already exists) are examples of proceduralism.** We put on a choreographed language dance and learn patterns different from our default ones.

Free writing and proceduralism are good opportunities for poetry. For new poetry writers, they are best practiced after gaining experience with **generative composing**, a term I use for a wide range of options between free writing and proceduralism (some of whose elements also crop up in generative composing). In other words, proceduralism – such as a sonnet with strictly rhymed lines, syllable counts, and regulated rhythm – is recommended for later developments in your poetry. Similarly, the challenge of writing "free verse" is more easily taken up once you have strengthened your writing muscles with the medial steps of generative composing.

Generative composing focuses not on the end product but on your compositional procedures and environments. Generative composing will release you, if you practice it conscientiously, from a treatment of the page as a "terra nullius" as well as from a focus on the end product of poetry. Staring at "blank" pages and worrying about whether we can write "good" poems gets in the way of poetry.

You can imagine the above spectrum in this way:

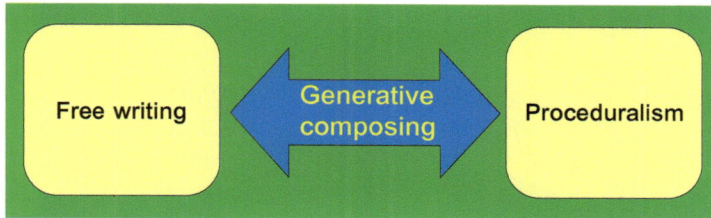

Figure 1. Composing spectrum

Two generative composing examples

These invented approaches do not focus on language "content," though some of my other generative composing strategies do. In these cases, the emphasis is on compositional structure.

Piling: Compose by writing one line then writing a line ABOVE that line, then writing another line ABOVE that line, and so on. Consider that you are piling up lines like flat rocks or plates, one atop the next. The poem composition might feel like air compression or like geological strata. The point is to disrupt habits of writing – in this case, the normative top-down approach – that can make you feel like you are supposed to get to a point. This relatively simple strategy can produce amazing line relations.

Jamming: Use only and frequent em dashes, the longest kind of dash, and question marks for punctuation. (The point is to disrupt habits of writing dominated by end-stopped sentences and declarative utterances.) Continue the compositional line: don't break the right margin, and rarely break to new sections. (The point here is to maximize line pressure in composing.) Here is an excerpt from "Cathedral," by Else von Freytag-Loringhoven, which resembles a jammed composition:

> Why didst thou go away from me?Say——why?art not enslaved by balmy
> wizzardryout of mine jewelled eye ?not by mine lips——so softly passionate——with
> harnessed strength——in bridled strain——musk——amber——myrrh and
> francincense——gold——damask——ivory——mine gothic cathedrál——is that
> upbuild in vainfor thee—— ?the whom I shall desire——to pray ?art nor thou
> worshipper nor devotee ?

2. Compose

This step is the most pleasurable, intense, and strict in its conditions. Once you have decided your generative approach, the aim is to compose as openly and expansively as possible. Compare it to having prepared fully for a long trek, with good shoes, a fine locale, and a large expanse of time: now you need to walk, letting go of everything except the full experience of the walk.

Let's say you choose to try **jamming**. You'll be ready with reams of paper, two pens (in case the first runs dry), or a computer screen free of everything except the expanded page-like view. You start at the bottom of a page and write a line such as "My lunchbox stares at breakfast's empty head": it doesn't matter where you start, because as you go UP the page the lines will enter into new relations with each other and you'll really enter the compositional event. So your first four lines, bottom up, might be:

4 when I stand up
3 a rivet-edge, a sigh the trees erase
2 a cleft idea merged
1 my lunchbox stares at breakfast's empty head

Four elements can help – I consider them crucial to success – with this composing step:

i. **Give yourself time.** Allow at least one hour of uninterrupted focus.

ii. **Maintain a willing presence toward language.** Fully inhabit and give yourself to the composition. Don't hesitate.

iii. **Create, don't evaluate.** If you critique while you are composing, you are not composing. Don't think: just write. Writing discovers the thoughts we have and brings them into form.

iv. **Write as much as you can.** Write expansively and keep going. Create as much writing as possible within your decided approach. This element is perhaps the most important of the four: as you exceed what you might have thought of as your compositional capacities, you enter more and more into regions of unprecedence, in other words into poetry. You get beyond your efforts to control and you enter into your ability to compose. Also, you need material in order to revise freely: you cannot revise what does not exist.

3. Revise

Revising your own poetry effectively can be as surprising and satisfying as finding yourself writing downside up. I'll start by emphasizing crucial revising moves then suggest other approaches I have found helpful.

i. Practice **poetic ecology**: first, save everything. Every version of the poem, every line you cut out. Put them in a file or a jar to bring out later, if and when you wish. New poetry writers should always save the Composing step in its entirety: don't save over your poem's first draft (at least, not until a year or so has passed). The other side of poetic ecology is being willing to **change anything** in the poem. Saving everything helps you feel free to let things go, because you know you can always get them back, re-make them, re-visit the energy of the first composition.

ii. **Print out your draft**. Revising (re-orienting, re-seeing, re-shaping) is partly accomplished with the visual body of your poem. The printed page is not the same body as the hand-written notebook or the illuminated screen. In this visually-oriented part of revising, imagine the poem is liquid: mobile, watery, or like a color and shape spectrum that you can pull one direction and another. When you have a substantial revision, print out that version of the poem too.

iii. **Read the poem out loud**. There is no substitute for this step: you need to revise with the ears of your mind. As with our living selves, the bodies of poems can arrive with, and can also be given in revision, a sensory intelligence that has a kind of living sufficiency: it's enough that sounds, enjambments, page layout, imagery, and the like are meaning in performance. In reading aloud, you hear and re-hear modulations, rhythms, tones, good moves and falterings from line to line. When you hear things like "wheel-spinning," for example, you can cut out the less interesting parts and retain the part that spins only one wheel beautifully for that moment of the poem.

iv. Articulate and foster the **affective center** of your poem. The affective center is a term I use for the predominant sense, feeling, or embodied mood of a poem. That mood can range from a specific feeling (righteous anger, for example) to an everyday generalized sense (perhaps a "slice of life") to a diaphanous focus on a sensory image. This central energy is particularly important to practice perceiving for a relatively short poem, something between 1-3 pages or so.

A note on "near" and "far" revising: if you have time after your composing step is complete (and saved), try immediately revising part or all of what you have written. Far revising happens when you allow some period of time – at least a week, ideally more than a month – between your composing step and your revising step.

While you save, print out, read out, and move around parts of your poem, below are some optional revision tactics to try.

i. Start with energy: go through your draft and find a line (or two) that jumps out in its sounds or image. Make that the start of the poem. Find a line in your draft that sounds good after that new beginning, and make it line 2 (or 3). Shift around subsequent lines accordingly.

ii. Exponentialize the energy between the poem's parts, whether between words or lines or sections. Exponentializing involves seeking a fruitful tension between definition and unresolvability, between determinate and nondeterminate meaning. In other words, sometimes the kitchen table spread should be riveted with tiny strawberries (relatively determinate description) and sometimes the magpies of your morning thought fly to a darkened room (relatively non-determinate meaning). Be ready to jump-cut, to put in blank lines between one section and another without worrying about how you got from one part to the next.

iii. End without closing meaning. Resolution-suspension helps the poem function as an event structure for meaning-making, allows the poem to breathe new life with every reading.

iv. Try different titles. Like a person's name, a title gives a handle to a poem. Sometimes it is effective to give a specific title (a date or place name, for example) to a somewhat abstruse poem and a less orienting title ("This poem loves you," for example) to a very specific poem. Some poems want no title at all.

Revision strategy example
In a longer version of teaching poetry revising, one of my approaches combines Extension, Rearrangement, Reorientation, and Resistance. Here is an example of a Rearrangement strategy.

Inversion
Sometimes the best revision strategy is to upend your draft. Starting with the last line and ending with the first line of your poem, write out the inversion completely. Such an inversion releases some of the resources of poetry from the kind of linear ("narrative" or "expository") impulses that dominate report writing. Inversion can be a great way to perceive the meaning-making energies of your draft composition.

Parting thoughts

Effective revision should help your poem generate meanings, where "meanings" includes feelings, sensations, mental work and play. The more you try to control a message in your poem, the less mental freedom your poem is allowed and the less it can deliver its meanings. This is a central paradox of art: you must give your poem a chance to glow in its place without restricting it to a single closed message. Poetry doesn't want to have only one meaning any more than we do.

For poetry to thrive, it needs you. You'll notice that textual poetry, of the digital and/or paper page, is the emphasis of this essay. There are many other ways to compose, present, and perform poetry. You can record yourself speaking, you can write centos and other appropriative assemblages, you can tattoo poetry on your body or perform poetry solo or with a group, spontaneously or in choreographed forms. You can code poetry or laser-stitch it into cellular membranes. You can blend poetry with other art forms: sound, sculpture, drawing, video, and more. Thankfully, imagination will always propose more ways to make poetry thrive for everyone.

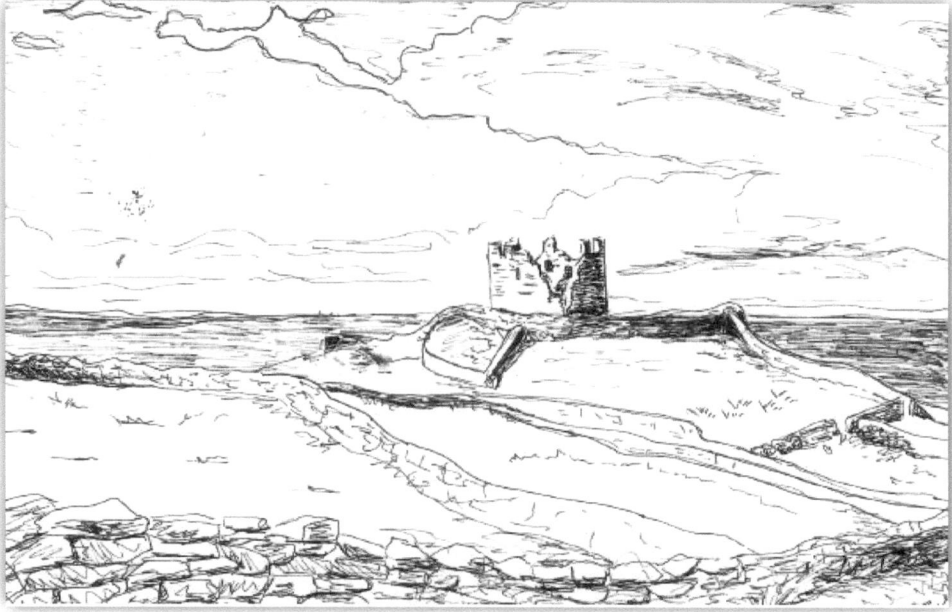

Aimee Vulinovich, Year 5. *Ruined church on the Aran Islands*. Fountain pen ink on paper, 2016. Series: Fountain pen sketches of significant places I have visited.

Rhythm, rhyme, simile and metaphor

Tanisha Jowsey

Lisa Samuel's chapter *Three Steps Towards Poetry* provides some great exercises for getting your poem on to the page and for ensuring that your ideas link together. Once you have some written ideas to edit, you might like to consider ways in which **rhythm** and **rhyme** feature in your poetry, as well as **similes** and **metaphors**. Attention to such devices can enhance your poem's capacity to evoke humour, emotions and imagination.

Rhythm

The way a poem sounds when you read it aloud, its heart beat, can critically shape your perception of that poem, in much the same way that the heartbeat of your patient can. Is the beat arrhythmic? Does it have a low ejection rate? Does the blood pump slowly through a long trudging valve, or does it gush and rush and skip frantically?

> Read this line out loud:
>
> Does the blood pump slowly through a long trudging valve, or does it gush and rush and skip frantically?

Notice how the words before the comma are slow to say and thus reinforce the subject of slowness. Notice how the words after the comma speed up. Using alliteration and onomatopoeia in poetry can be useful toward informing the rhythm of your poem.

You may also recall from your high school days in English class that some poems have procedural didactic rhythms, such as the iambic pentameter. This means that the rhythm is predictable. Iambic pentameter, for example, looks like this:

De da – de da – de da– de da– de da

De da – de da – de da– de da– de da

A haiku, in contrast, is a three-line poem that has five syllables for the first line, then seven for the second line, and five syllables for the third line. It may look more like this:

De – da – de – da – de

de – da – de – da – de – da -de

de – da – de – da – de

Similarly, some syllables may predictably begin with hard consonants or soft vowels, or simply hidden in the middle of a word. So depending on the chosen words, your haiku might actually look more like this:

De da – de – da de

de – da – da – da de da – de

de da – de – da de

Here is an example of a haiku I wrote (27):

<u>Haiku III</u>

The scent so striking

soft purple leaves inviting

fleeting like my youth.

De – da – de – da de

de – da de – da – de da de

de da – de – da – de

A predictable rhythm can be very soothing for the reader and can offer the poem a sense of flow. This can be particularly effective in romantic or melancholic poetry. Disruption to an established rhythm can be just as effective. It can alert the reader to a change in the subject matter and can create a sense of urgency or even alarm. So it is worth having a look at your poem's rhythm and checking whether it is reinforcing or at odds with the message you are conveying.

Time, slime, crime and rhyme

Rhyme can function in a similar way to rhythm by creating a sense of predictability and flow. If you are considering using rhyme in your poem it can be very useful to first write the draft of the poem that does not rhyme, so that you can establish a strong storyline or message without the complications that rhyme can add. When we are new to writing poetry we can easily slip into cliché and stereotypes and superficial-sounding poetry by rhyming. We find a word that rhymes and although it carries a different meaning from our intention we pop it in any way for the sake of rhyming. The reader is left wondering, what does time and slime and crime have to do with rhyme? Such oddities almost always have the unwanted effect of distancing the reader from the heart of your poem.

If you are creating poetry as a demonstration of your critical reflection then this kind of distancing outcome can be disastrous.

However, this book includes multiple examples of critically reflective poetry where rhyme has been used effectively to support the predictability and flow of the poem. The poems of Josh Coulter, Anna Perera, Demi Poynter, and Hannah Smiley included in this collection, are great examples of the message being supported by both rhythm and rhyme.

Which words in your poem are the most critical?

Here is a strategy I use to identify the important words and allow other words to change/be replaced to facilitate rhyme.

Below is a poem I wrote called Pet of Ten Years (27), where rhythm and rhyme feature. Most of the poem follows a common rhyme pattern:

a, b, c, b   (this is a common pattern in a four-line rhyming stanza).

The middle stanza follows a different pattern; the first two lines do not rhyme while the remaining five lines do.

When I wrote this poem I thought about the message I was trying to convey, that my dog – who had been the centre of my world for so long – might be ignored once my baby was born. I wanted this message to be strong in the final lines of the poem. Therefore I wrote those lines first, "but you won't even see me there —— as you rock your sleeping bub." Then I wrote 'up' the two lines before them; "come six o'clock I'll look to you —— for the daily walk then grub." By writing the lines in this order I was able to ensure that the final lines were strong and that I wasn't left trying to find a rhyming word for my (important) final line. I did not want to risk having an altered meaning on that final line for the sake of rhyme. Rather, I moved that risk higher up in the poem and had to find a word that rhymed with "bub."

Why didn't I use the word baby? Aside from there not being many options that rhyme with baby, I wanted the character of the dog to come through and colloquial words like bub and grub seemed more effective towards supporting that character development.

```
PET OF TEN YEARS

I feel nothing, I replied
but the dog believed me not.
Nothing is a myth, a luxury
your mind decays with rot.

Listen up!
He chastised me
hear the tone in my woof
these next eight months of growth
are going to be tough.
Feeling nothing is not enough.
Feeling nothing is but a myth.

Admit it now, his tail twitched
you feel everything and yearn
I'll be replaced before too long
as your feelings grow and churn
come six o'clock I'll look to you
for the daily walk then grub
but you won't even see me there
as you rock your sleeping bub.
```

Finally, and in returning to the former section on rhythm, *Pet of Ten Years* provides a clear example of how the rhythm is disrupted with **"Listen up!"**

Similes and metaphors

A simile is a comparison between two things that (often at first seem very different and unconnected, but) share something in common. For example, "the decrepit fence hung from the post like an old man from his cane." The simile encourages us to think of the fence and the old man as sharing a common thread. The thread is not always clearly spelled out and this allows room for the readers own interpretations to surface based on their personal experiential knowledge of fences, old men, canes, and so forth. The reader may interpret the commonality to be that of dependence, both the fence and the old man are dependent on something else to stand erect. Likewise, the reader may see the common thread in terms of age, ageing and decay. The simile can therefore serve to raise more than one thread of commonality between two seemingly disparate things/objects/concepts/emotions.

A metaphor is when one thing is described as being something else. It is "a figure of speech in which a word or phrase is applied to an object or action to which it is not literally applicable"; "a thing regarded as representative or symbolic of something else."(28)

> Gather ye rosebuds while ye may;
>
> Old Time is still a-flying:
>
> And this same flower that smiles today
>
> Tomorrow will be dying.
>
> -Robert Herrick, To the Virgins, to make much of time

For example, **"Beware of jealousy, my lord! It's a green-eyed monster that makes fun of the victims it devours,"** from William Shakespeare's *Othello*(29). Jealousy (an emotion) *is* a monster (a mythical creature associated with fear and danger). In my view, the metaphor is a more assertive poetic device than the simile. It leaves less room for the reader to draw their own associations and conclusions. Metaphors have been used effectively in poetry to map two conceptual domains.(30) Some metaphors take the form of an underlying conceptual mapping; *A is a B* (such as Bob **Dylan's "Time is a jet plane, it moves too fast."** Others are more extended or allegorical, such as **"Two roads diverged in a wood, and I – – I took the one less travelled by, – And that has made all the difference,"** by Robert Frost (30) or Robert Herrick's *To the Virgins, to make much of time,* where virgins are likened to flowers.

When reading through your poem ask yourself these kinds of questions:

- **What is the most important element in this part of the poem?**
- **What is this […] like?**
- **If this […] that I'm writing about were something else, what would it be?**
- **What experience have I had that was similar to this one or informed how I feel about this one?**
- **Could this section of the poem be more effective if I used a different metaphor/word/sound/pause instead?**

As Lisa Samuels has suggested in the previous chapter, it is a good idea to keep all drafts of your poems so that you can feel free to make changes without the fear of losing anything. Try different metaphors out for the same section of poem. Write the same section of your poem as a simile and as a metaphor – read them both out loud. Which one sounds better? Which one do you feel more comfortable with?

Ask yourself: does this simile/metaphor add anything to the poem? Is it necessary? Does it evoke emotion or imagination? Does it move the story deeper?

Is it too cryptic?

Asking and responding to these kinds of reflective editing questions can be really helpful towards improving your poem's ability to engage the reader on multiple levels. Robert Sullivan's poem *King Tawhiao's Garden,* provides a wonderful example of imagery and metaphor working together to create a sense of tension between history and freedom.

King Tawhiao's Garden

The entrance to the king's food garden

was the old tree surrounded by carvings

on Pukekawa, opposite Auckland Museum,

where he defended the city

from the great tribes to the north.

I am but a dolphin diving in the backdrop

of this tree, swimming through the earth.

- Robert Sullivan, Poetry NZ, Yearbook 2, Nov 2015, Issue 50

Foreign body in the operating room

Tanisha Jowsey

What follows is a writing exercise that I engaged in under the wonderful direction of Selina Tusitala Marsh at a creative writing workshop in December 2016 that was hosted by Helen Sword of the Centre for Learning and Research in Higher Education. Participants were asked to write about their project/topic of interest for twenty minutes. After this initial writing phase participants were asked to only use what we had already written to form a poem. We had seven minutes to identify six lines in what we had written, that were each 1-7 words long. Thus, in less than half an hour we created a first draft of a poem. In the weeks that followed, I refined the poem that emerged from the writing workshop and it is presented here below the original 20-minute text.

Is narrative medicine just for doctors and nurses? Might medical anthropologists and others also have a place in narrative medicine?

When I awoke this morning I could already feel the familiar nervous beast in my puku. I dressed, kissed my sleeping baby, and marched in the dark to my car.
Arriving now at the hospital, 6am, feels foreign to me. I cross the road along with others already dressed in their scrubs. I greet my research colleague Jane and we wait in the brightly lit corridor near the large glass doors. Patients and families also wait here. People speak in hushed whispers sporadically as though cautiously filling the space. I can smell their fears, I can taste them.
Or are they my own?
The anaesthetic consultant opens the door. "Change in there. We are in O.R. Three. Suzie will show you."
Jane and I enter the changing room. Closets, clothes, bags, shoes, shelves. Scrubs are stacked in piles from smallest to largest. Jane is smaller than me. She is half my size. Her Facebook profile picture looks like it was pulled from a Vogue magazine. Mine doesn't. Self-conscious, and reminded of school days in the changing rooms, I reach for the 'XL' top and quickly change clothes. This top is *miles* too big for me but I've already touched it.
Have I contaminated it?

I look silly and I know it.

We speak nervously about nothing.

A nurse, presumably Suzie, enters to hurry us along. "Hats, booties, masks there, help yourself." She says this with her back to us and a finger pointing to a shelf loaded with unfamiliar small boxes and artefacts from a culture that is not my own.

Bustling and busy; the operating staff weave seamlessly through the space, talking in relaxed tones and joking about a television show. I scramble into the mask and tie blue bootie laces over my shoes. Jane follows my lead. White walls. White doors. We enter Theatre Three.

The patient, a large man in his sixties, lies on the bed, speaking nervously about nothing. His blood pressure is high. I wonder how high mine is. A nurse pushes a trolley into position. "Don't stand there," she barks. I move. "No, not there, you're blocking the emergency doors."

I squash my body against the window. I am a fly. A speck of dust. A micro-something that nobody need notice.

The anaesthetist enters and walks straight over to me. "Hi Tanisha, those are hats on your feet and your mask is on inside out."

I look down.

Oh crap.

Those are not booties.

The anaesthetist speaks to the nurse about instruments while I turn maroon and swallow the lump of embarrassment.

This is not how I expected my first day in theatre to go. I'm a chief investigator. I'm a medical anthropologist. I have seen E.R., Scrubs, and Chicago Hope. How did I miss the clues that could help me fit in?

I am a foreign body. Even the patient is dressed appropriately!

I feel very very small.

"It's an easy mistake to make," Jane says with kind eyes.

After fixing my attire I introduce myself to the patient. Jane listens and watches attentively. We smile. The patient tells us of his children while they find a line. And now he sleeps. A nurse whizzes in and before I know what is happening she catheterizes him. I look away; embarrassed to see his vulnerability. The skull is opened. I see his brain. Blood drips into the steel bucket. The smell of burned flesh grips my nostrils. Oh no. I'm going to vomit. I feel the rush of heat to my head. I'm sweating. Now cold. Oh God. I can't bear another embarrassment here. I quickly reach for the door handle and head past the scrubbing basins out into the corridor.

Cold air catches me.

I breathe.

Thank heavens. I'm going to be okay.

At the basin I splash cold water on my face and breathe slowly. Deeply.

I return to the site. The surgeon looks up, his hand in someone's head.

"I didn't think you were coming back."

I very nearly wasn't.

It is a strange and foreign culture. I'm there to study communication, power, hierarchies, teamwork, and how people cope in high stress situations. It is important towards informing patient safety. These snazzy words look great on grant applications. But the reality of the OR is not captured in those words. I'm not an authority in this space. I'm just standing nearby, trying not to stand out, trying to make sense of it all.

Reflections

Snazzy words on grant applications

mean nothing in this place.

I see a patient vulnerable

fear lines his pulse and face.

Operating theatre dynamics

mean nothing in my state.

I see myself vulnerable

hats and mask to contemplate.

-Tanisha Jowsey

Aimee Vulinovich, Year 5. *Bethells Beach, West Auckland*. Fountain pen ink on

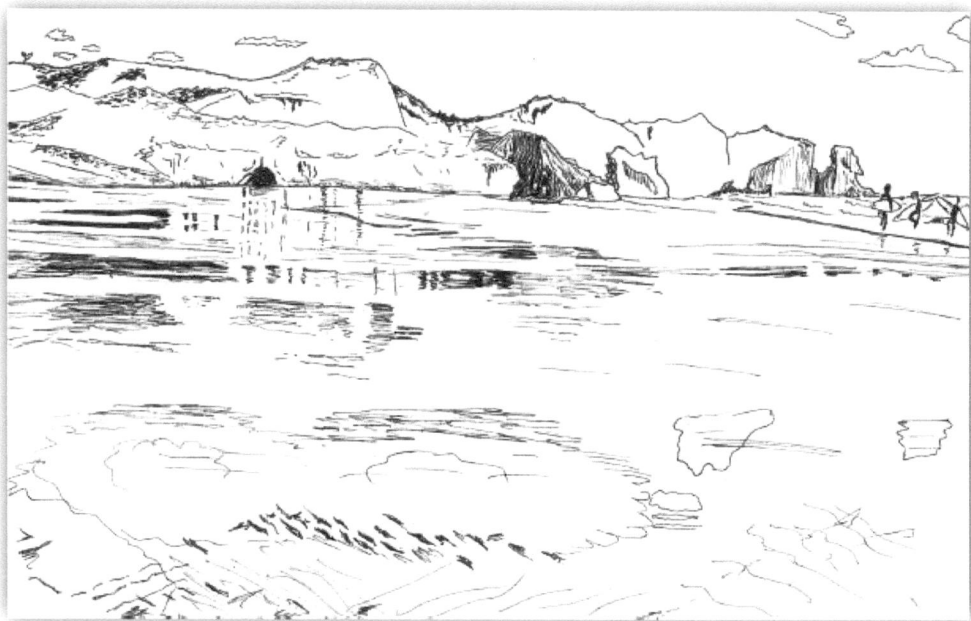

paper, 2016. Series: Fountain pen sketches of significant places I have visited.

Art composition – strategies to try while creating art

Tanisha Jowsey

In 2016, twenty-five visual art works were put forward by students as part of their Portfolios. The diversity in these works – from sketch pad anatomical illustrations to water colour landscapes – demonstrated that even when limited to visual art the options for where to take it are endless. As with poetry, the strategies used to strengthen the art pieces ranged in complexity and skill.

In this chapter I focus on some of the artistic strategies that the new-to-art or emerging artist might like to try in order to strengthen their skills. The strategies concerning critical reflection are largely the same as with any of the critical reflection writing; they are intellectual and emotion-engaged. They require that the artist think deeply and attentively to the message they want to convey and the strategies they will utilise to support that message.

If you want the critically-reflective focus of your art work to be an oxygen mask, for example, then it can be useful to first start with a pen and paper and workshop a few different ways of presenting the mask to ensure that it will remain the point of focus when you've completed the image.

Drawing

Drawing consists of lines.

At first glance this sentence seems simple enough, even blatantly obvious. However, there is vast complexity and a multiple array of outcomes emergent from the different shapes, lengths, hardness, thickness, and angles of lines.

Here's an exercise to illustrate:

Drawing a tree

On a blank piece of plain paper draw the same tree a few times, using these line techniques:

1. With a single line (don't take your pen off the page) draw the whole tree
2. Draw a tree by only using lines that all head in the same direction
3. Draw a tree with a thick point pen and with a fine point pen
4. Try cross-hatching lines as a means of exploring shadow or adding depth to the image

5. Draw a tree with as few lines as possible then move the paper and draw the tree again using as few lines as possible. The second tree may overlap with the first tree. Move the paper again and draw a third tree. And so on. This can create the basis for a multi-layered collage of trees. You might then choose to colour in particular overlapping line sections.
6. Try making the image appear three dimensional by adding vanishing lines and a vanishing point
7. Draw a horizon line. This grounds objects and creates distance
8. Try making one part of the drawing busy with many lines and one part of the image vacant of lines to create contrast and/between points of focus
9. Try drawing in different mediums, with chalk, pastels, ink, felt pens or charcoal. Some of these mediums smudge and blend to blur or soften lines (in which case it can be helpful to use hair spray or a fine art spray for cementing the drawing and preventing further accidental smudging).

You now have a few drawings of a tree. Notice how the different line techniques contribute to the overall feel of the tree. Which of these techniques might best support the idea you wish to convey?

In addition to these line techniques you may want to look at a few 'how to draw ...' books/apps/videos/magazines.

Space and colour

When you begin your drawing a good option is to start with ruling up the border. This gives you a clear idea of how much space you have to work within. Once you have established clarity in what it is that you want to draw/convey you might like to consider how the use of space can help you to achieve that focus. If, for example, you want the message to be about the importance of cats to your health and wellbeing, you might want the image of the cat to take centre stage. To achieve this, you can literally draw a cat in the middle of the space. The cat might take up all of the space. Or it might take up one-ninth of the space (since humans tend to look along grids of nine to establish 'beauty' in images, including photography and art works).

Another way to think about emphasizing the point of focus would be to use light/dark and/or colour to accentuate it. A small white cat in a busy page of grey objects can be a good way of accentuating the point of focus. This technique was effectively applied in the film *Schindler's List*, where the audience was drawn to follow the movements of a small girl in a red jacket amidst an otherwise grey scape.

Cartoon illustrations

You don't have to be born with a crayon in your hand to be able to create constructive and effective cartoon illustrations. Most of us have memories of drawing throughout our childhood, in a cartoonish kind of way (and some of us never stopped).

Here are some examples of how complex ideas can be portrayed quickly and effectively through cartoon illustrations.

Tribe theatre uses light and colour to emphasise the different surgical, anaesthetic and nursing teams of the operating theatre, which Weller, Boyd & Cumin refer to as 'tribes.' (31) They explain that siloed approaches to care do not serve the patient's safety and health outcomes as well as integrated approaches do. Weller et al. identify several strategies to inform the creation of a single operating theatre tribe, including information sharing and shared mental models through the use of structured communication models. They write, "[w]ith increasing complexity and even more specialisation of skills, the current healthcare environment demands effective communication and teamwork to reliably deliver best patient care." (31)

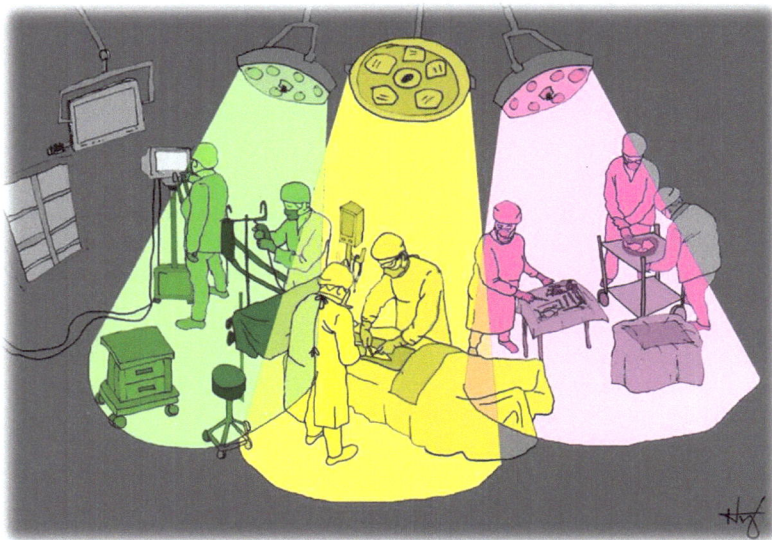

Image detail: Hugh Brocklebank. *Tribe Theatre.* Developed for the Centre for Medical and Health Sciences Education. The University of Auckland. 2015.

To draw this kind of cartoon the illustrator needs a basic knowledge of operating theatres – of clothing, how space is utilised, technology in the theatre, and so forth. The level of detail needed to convey the message is often very different from the level of detail used to depict the style of the cartoon.

Doctor Valiant uses a basic drawing style to demonstrate the idea that the doctor is often willing to do whatever it takes to fight off death, even when death of the patient is inevitable. It raises a question around when the doctor should put down his metaphorical sword.

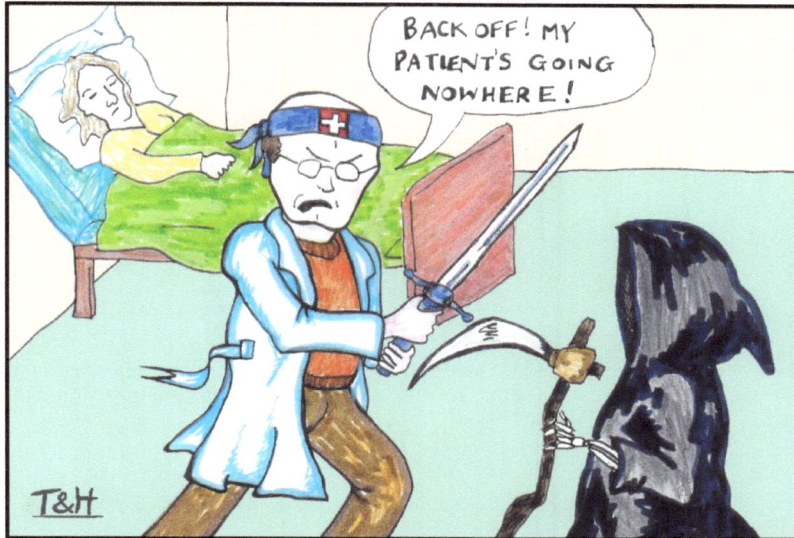

Image detail: Hugh Brocklebank and Tanisha Jowsey. *Doctor Valiant.* Developed for the Medical School, Australian National University. 2012.

As with *Doctor Valiant, Money Bag* (on the following page) draws on metaphor to illustrate the message. For the metaphor to work effectively in imagery it helps when you provide the viewer with as many clues as possible to surround the metaphor. In this case, the viewer can see that the hospital bed has a large sack of money where they would typically expect to see a patient. The speech bubble further supports the metaphor by telling us that the money bag is actually somebody's dying grandmother. This is again supported by the legal will. All of these clues work together to explore the concept that the decision to turn off life support for a critically ill patient may sometimes be informed by factors beyond those of the patient's likelihood of recovering.

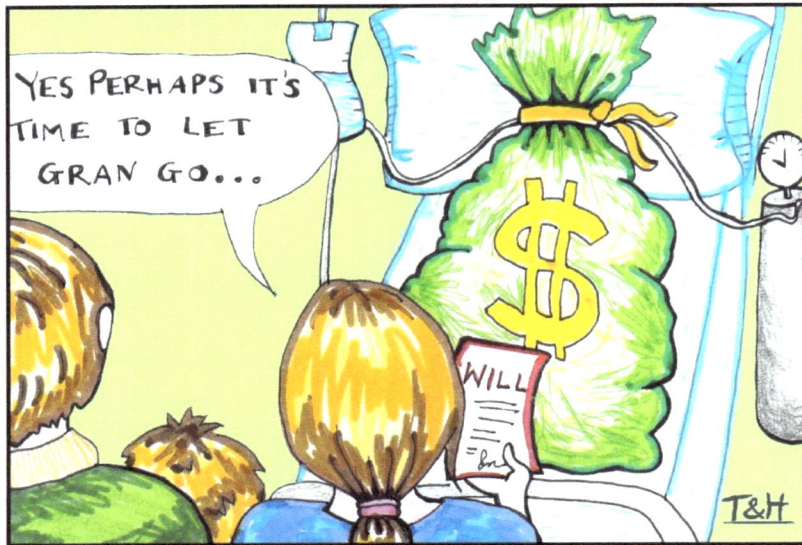

Image detail: Hugh Brocklebank and Tanisha Jowsey. *Money Bag*. Developed for the Medical School, Australian National University. 2012.

Cartoons can be a great deal of fun to think about and draw. Much of the hard work is with coming up with an idea of how to convey your message. Don't be afraid to experiment with the idea; depict the same image from different angles. If you have difficulty drawing particular things, like hands, then workshop ways in which you can draw the image and make the hands easiest to draw or hidden from view.

Painting

I'm not much of a drawer, I'm a painter and a sculptor. As you can see from cartoons above that I have worked on with Hugh Brocklebank, being good at drawing is not entirely necessary, you just have to be good enough to convey the message (for example, I'm drawing a cat, I want my audience to be able to tell that it's a cat). The rest is icing and cherries.

I feel much more comfortable painting. Whether its water colour, oil or acrylic, I'm having fun. The easiest medium of these three is acrylic. It is reasonably inexpensive, full-bodied, flexible, and dries quickly. If you want to make a painting that will last for a hundred years then don't add water to the acrylic paint as it makes the paint more brittle and also reduces its vibrancy. Instead, use an acrylic drying retarder product from your local fine arts store. If the hundred year trajectory isn't top of your priorities then by all means experiment with water in the mix.

Here are two pieces of my own art that I share with you as an opportunity for us to explore *process* and *self-appraisal*. Both can be useful to consider when creating art, and can be especially useful in terms of critical reflection.

Example 1: colour, shape and simplicity

Here's a finger painting I did in 2011 for friends in Europe.

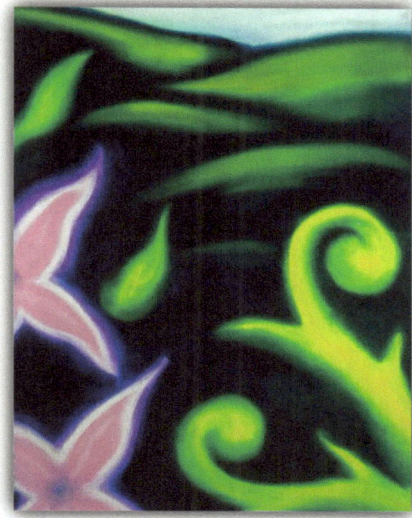

This piece was painted in oils on unstretched primed canvas, it is called *Memories of New Zealand*.

Process: To create it I first thought about what I wanted my message to be, the colours I wanted to use and the shapes that could reinforce my message. I used a light HB pencil to draw some rough guide lines onto the canvas. I drew them lightly because often the pencil lines can still be seen in the final product (this is especially so when using watercolour paint). I was mindful that I did not want the painting to be too busy, because that busy-ness would be at odds with the message. I chose oil sticks to paint with because they are flexible and have a reasonably fast drying time (overnight). I used cotton tips to aid the creation of sharp corners on the flower petals. The painting took about 30 minutes to complete.

Self-appraisal: I like the simplicity of the piece. It felt enjoyable to blend the yellows and blues with my index finger. The flowers don't work. They are too non-specific. What kind of flower is this? How do I know it's from New Zealand and not somewhere else? I could have worked harder on that part of the painting. I could have workshopped that a bit more, left it to dry and gone over it with a wash, or increased/changed the detail to strengthen that element in the painting. Overall, it is relaxing and inviting to look at and it reminds me of the countryside where I grew up in New Zealand (although the hills are really only that green in winter).

Example 2: layers

The final piece is called *Wai Tai,* from the Imagined Realities collection, ANCA Gallery, Canberra, Australia, June 2008.

Wai Tai

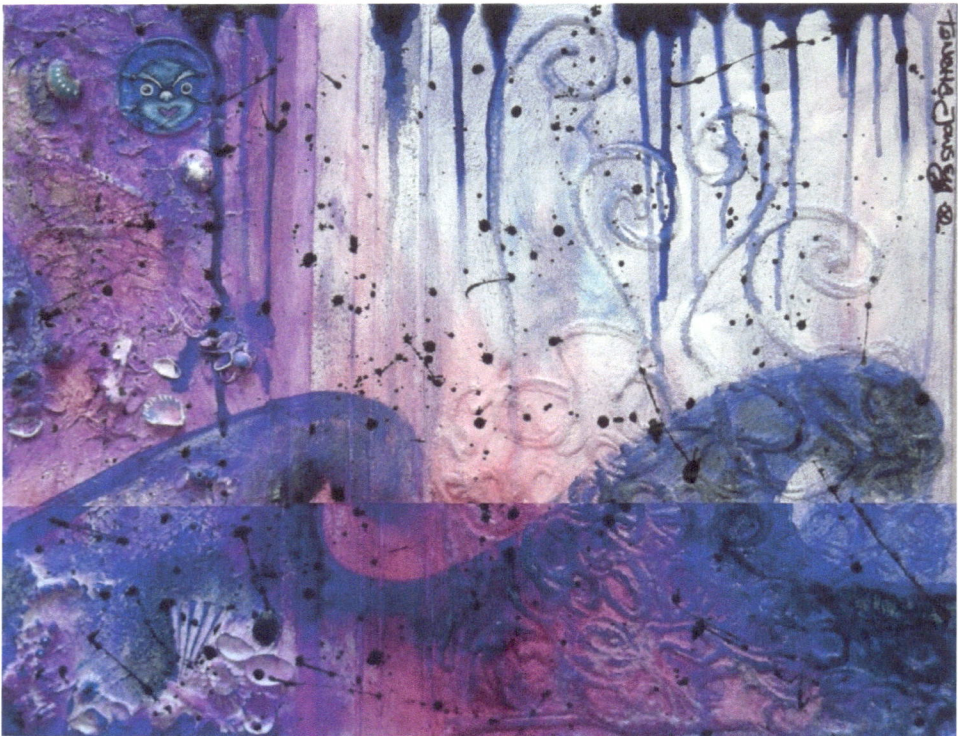

Wai Tai explores salt water spirits in New Zealand waters. It is mixed media on stretched canvas.

Process: This painting explores layers. First I played with glue, flicking, swirling, dripping and globbing PVA wood glue over the primed wall paper that I had previously stuck onto the stretched canvas. Once that was dry I used a heavy moulding structure gel to embed shells and dried seaweeds that I had collected from a New Zealand beach. Once that was dry I began dripping variously thinned acrylic paints on. Then I painted the background colours and waves and water taniwha. Finally, I flicked and splattered navy acrylic paint over top. The process took several days to account for drying time.

Self appraisal: I love this piece. It feels watery and the many layers create a sense of depth and movement. I enjoyed the process of creating it and the final product is a pleasure to look at and to touch. Because of the multiple textures this piece works as sensory art for blind audiences too. As my Grandmother was unwell when I created this, and died shortly thereafter, I donated it to the Palliative wing of the RedCliffe Hospital in Brisbane, where she was cared for in her final days.

James Corbett's untitled piece of the anatomical sketch over a layer of Maori designs (in the Health and Wellbeing section of this book) provides a strong example of how layering can be used effectively to enhance complexity, aesthetics, and depth.

Marvellous painting tips

Colour counts: A painting almost always looks more impressive if it's on a coloured background. The most striking backgrounds to choose are red and black. So if your painting skills fall short of the Da Vinci level you might like to try painting onto a coloured back ground. You can do this by painting on coloured card or by doing a plain coloured wash over your canvas before you start with the rest of the painting.

Colour counts: pale colours, pastel colours, yellows and warm oranges and pinks are calming to view. Monet provides us with plenty of examples to illustrate. Strong bold uninterrupted colours can stir stronger emotions in us. Paintings that explore emotions such as anger, depression and danger are often well-supported by colours that can create such emotions in the first instance.

Paint the background first and the foreground last. The order of painting can be detected in the final image and can inform how the audience sees depth.

Give a painting time. Leave it to bubble away in your mind for a while then return to your canvas with fresh ideas. Acrylic changes colour slightly from wet to dry. It can be worthwhile to leave the paint to dry and to look at it under natural light to see what the paint is doing.

Always **mix more colour** than you think you will need (because it's hard to recreate an exact match, and darn near impossible if you are working in acrylic and the first batch has run out and dried already).

Layers are fabulous. They add depth to your work. You might like to start with a mixture of thinned out paint and a wide brush. Leave the first layer to dry. Choose a different colour or brush and add another layer. Leave it to dry. Try a slightly thicker mixture of paint and run it thick along one side of the canvas then turn the canvas on its edge to encourage the paint to run/drip down, try jiggling the canvas a little. You could even get a straw and blow on the paint to move it in different directions. Try cutting out some pictures from magazines and sticking them onto the canvas. Try drawing over top of the magazine images and layers. Glue on some gold leaf or even an actual leaf from the tree outside. Paint onto the leaf. Stick on some fluff. The possibilities are endless (and it's jolly good fun).

Have fun. If you are not enjoying the process, if it's just not working for whatever reason, then stop. Take a break. Return to it later. Or start again.

Go easy on yourself. There is nothing wrong with ceremoniously burning art that just didn't work. Indeed, there is nothing wrong with unceremoniously burning it. But sometimes it is nice to keep it as a memoir, even if it didn't turn out how you expected it would, or how you would have liked it to. Art is a subjective and intersubjective journey. Go easy on yourself. We artists are all learning and exploring, always.

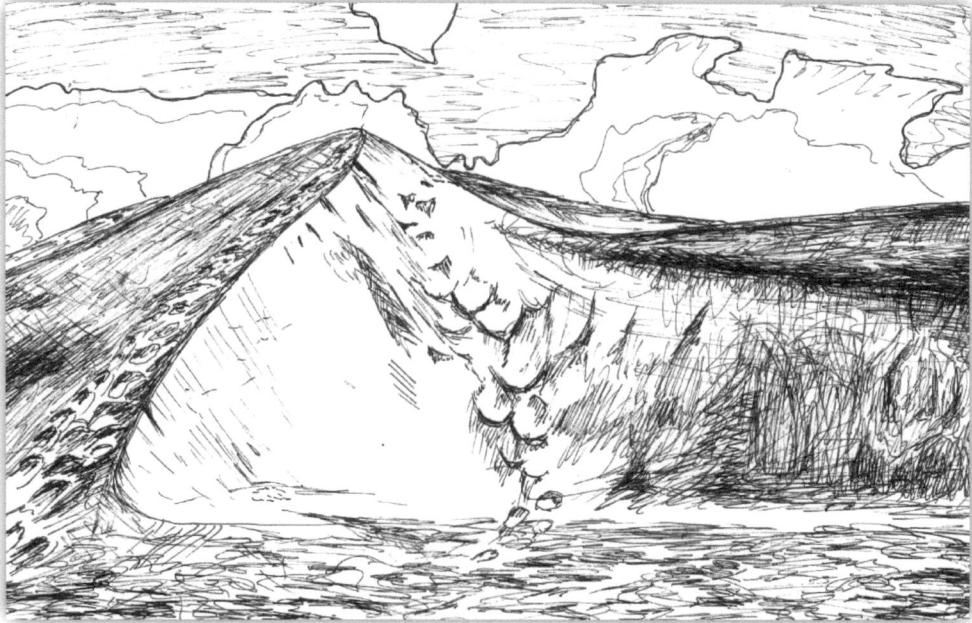

Aimee Vulinovich, Year 5, *Bethells Lake, Sand Dunes*. Fountain pen ink on paper, 2016. Series: Fountain pen sketches of significant places I have visited.

Poetry and art assessment for inclusion in this collection: process

Tanisha Jowsey

The works presented here have gone through a review process, where they were appraised by a team of university faculty (Tanisha Jowsey, Jill Yielder, Sharyn Esteves, Art Nahill, Rachael Yielder) based on the following evaluative rubric:

- Overall message: poor-average-strong-impressive
- Critical reflection: poor-average-strong-impressive
- Development of empathy: poor-average-strong-impressive

- Poetry: Successful use of poetic devices: poor-average-strong-impressive
- Poetry: words are moving/engaging: poor-average-strong-impressive

- Visual art: Artistic merit: poor-average-strong-impressive
- Visual art: image is moving/engaging: poor-average-strong-impressive

This assessment criteria is different to that of the PPS Portfolios.

The rubric speaks to quality of engagement with the subject material and critical reflection; including through development of empathy, which is a key element in narrative medicine. We noticed that few poems scored 'impressive' in Development of empathy and Successful use of poetic devices. Development of empathy may be an area worthy of future research in terms of narrative medicine and of our student portfolios.

Many of the 2016 students who submitted poetry or art as part of their portfolio submitted more than one piece, with some students submitting as many as seven poems or five visual art pieces.

Students whose pieces scored 'impressive' or 'strong' on the rubric were invited to contribute, and most of those students who were invited to contribute their works accepted the invitation (89 poems and 13 art pieces are included). Pieces that scored lower on the rubric were discussed by the committee to reach a decision on whether or not to invite the student to submit the work for this collection.

We are delighted that so many invited students chose to submit and celebrate their works.

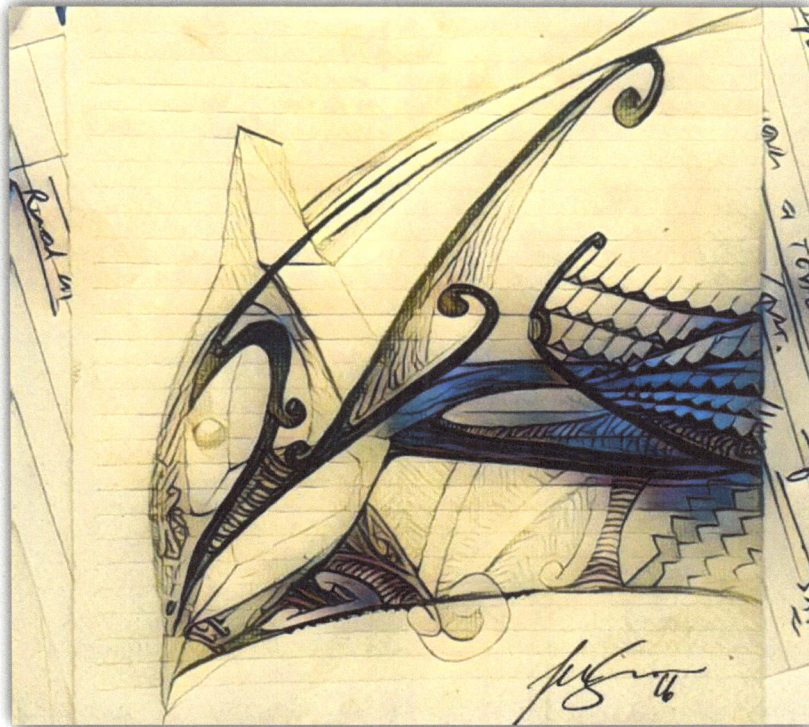

Coll Campbell, Year 4. *Tui Forest Lore*, 2016, (Front cover)

Creative context

An original graphically rendered sketch of a native New Zealand Tui bird (Prosthemadera novae zealandiae) on Auckland City Hospital clinical note paper. I have placed it on the title page because of the connection I have found in Maori folklore and how its mythical symbolism reflects the modern and historical role of the doctor. This connection is best surmised by the following quote;

> *"this bird can claim an exalted lineage and a semi-divine origin, inasmuch as it originated with one Parauri, one of the offspring of the Earth Mother and Sky Parent; likewise this Parauri was one of three guardians appointed in times remote to preserve the welfare and fertility of the forest, as also of its occupants"*

> *- Best, 1977, p. 292 (32).*

Concluding thoughts

Tanisha Jowsey

This collection began as a conversation between a few teachers in the PPS Domain that celebrated the diversity, quality and unpretentious depictions of experience that our medical students present in their Portfolios. Twelve months later we have a collection to celebrate. To study and practice medicine is no small thing. It can be relentlessly demanding. It can offer health care practitioners experiences that bring into sharp focus harsh injustices and inequities in health, while also offering them experiences of feeling that one person's caring attention can make a world of difference. We have seen such realisations come to life in the works presented here. Harry Alexander's *A forgotten promise,* for example, explores it in terms of cultural inequity:

> Crowded houses | A feeding ground for illness | And for inequities to grow | That a sore throat could cause | So much hurt | Who could know? | History repeats itself.

Others have explored the divide between the biomedical gaze and socio-cultural facets. T.J. Mitchell's poem *Programming Error* is a fine example of how the student can recall with such vibrancy the experience of exploring a patient's chest cavity, lungs and bronchus but fails to recall the patient's name. Similarly, in Natasha Trilokekar's poem *Of course*, she writes:

> It's an adult incontinence product, Mr. Surgeon. | Not a diaper, nor a bib, not a cot or a crib, | But then she is not your mother.
> She is 302. | Left Hip Arthroplasty under General Anaesthesia with Desflurane, | Nil by Mouth, No Known Allergies, Does not require return of body parts. | Oh good, one less bloody form to fill.

Another insightful example comes from Sarah Shirley's *Poor Historian*, where the patient is referred to as a poor historian because his medical history is so poor, which is then expertly contrasted with his rich social engagement and recollection of his morning's activities. Additionally, the character development in this poem is beautifully constructed and contributes to our sense of empathy with the patient:

> last night was sweaty and hot | Funny for this time of year, right doc? | Ate five weetybix things with milk, lots of sugar | but then my tummy felt funny, did some big burps, | frightened the tuis squabbling in the kowhai tree.

Indeed, much of the poetry throughout this collection depicts tender moments where a single word, touch or look connects with the writer in a way that encourages them to think more empathetically towards the patient specifically, and towards patients and their family members in general. Holly Wilson's poem *Acceptance* captures this in attention to nervousness, memory and association:

> you won't remember me | fumbling with my hands
> … as I inserted a small needle | into your well mapped skin
> … but you took my hand and told me | "you young thing, you are doing so well – | I am so proud of you"
> … and how a weight felt lifted off my shoulders.

In her poem *Nameless*, Tilisi Puloka writes:

> My husband is watching, please be gentle | He can't see me like this | …because it's the last time.

Here the student explores empathy through the depiction of an old woman who is nearing death. Many of the poems in the Health & Wellbeing section also tackle issues of death and dying. Students explore the fragility of life and the sacredness of a 'good death.' They also explore the frustrations of realising the limits of medicine; bringing our attention back to the injustices of health.

The art works that students put forward for this collection, although fewer in number, are equally rich in aesthetic qualities and engagement with the PPS domain. Aimee Vulinovich's sketches of places around the Auckland region speak to her experiences outside of medical school. They have a meditative quality, as does Joanna Davie's painting of *Takou Bay*, Northland. Demi Poynter's piece *Meant to write reflection but I coloured* in instead also holds this meditative relaxing quality.
Freya Forstner's sketch *Whia* explores age and time in a beautiful solemn portrait of an old Maori woman. Whia is a Maori word meaning 'how long' and is used to explore duration, such as age and ageing. The audience is invited to consider longevity and ageing of the depicted woman, and of themselves. This is in stark contrast to Coll Campbell's *Self-portrait*, as a happy, energetic, young, fit doctor in scrubs. The bright colours and fun style chosen in this piece support a message that Coll is enthusiastic about his profession. Similarly, Hannah Smiley's *Daisies* presents us with a feeling of hope through the subject material and use of light.

Overall, the poems and art presented here have taken us on a journey of critical reflection about medicine as a profession and about health and wellbeing of patients, whanau, friends, doctors, medical students, and people from all walks of life. As individual pieces – and collectively – they encourage us to think deeply about a specific issue or experience. We wonder how we might respond in a similar situation, they remind us of our own experiences, and they offer us hope that our students who will soon be doctors do care and do have insight into the importance of health, wellbeing, empathy, professionalism, ethics, and people.

Let's conclude, in gratitude and hope, with this Maori proverb (33):

He aha te mea nui o te ao
What is the most important thing in the world?

He tangata, he tangata, he tangata
It is the people, it is the people, it is the people.

Reference list

1. Yielder J, Moir F. Assessing the Development of Medical Students' Personal and Professional Skills by Portfolio. Journal of Medical Education and Curricular Development. 2016(3):9-15.
2. Rapport N. Transcendent Individual: Towards a Literary and Liberal Anthropology. . London and New York: Routledge; 1997.
3. Kamhi MM. Who Says That's Art?: A Commonsense View of the Visual Arts. Pro Arte Books; 2014.
4. Frank AW. The wounded storyteller: Body, illness, and ethics. University of Chicago Press; 2013.
5. Charon R. Narrative medicine: a model for empathy, reflection, profession, and trust. Jama. 2001;286(15):1897-902.
6. Ahlzén R. The doctor and the literary text—potentials and pitfalls. Medicine, health care and philosophy. 2002;5(2):147-55.
7. Charon R. Narrative medicine: Honoring the stories of illness. 2006.
8. Miller E, Balmer D, Hermann MN, Graham MG, Charon R. Sounding narrative medicine: Studying students' professional identity development at Columbia University College of Physicians and Surgeons. Academic medicine: journal of the Association of American Medical Colleges. 2014;89(2):335.
9. Greenhalgh T, Hurwitz B. Narrative Based Medicine Dialogue and discourse in clinical practice. 1998.
10. Greenhalgh T. Narrative based medicine in an evidence based world. BMJ. 1999;318(7179):323-5.
11. DasGupta S, Charon R. Personal illness narratives: using reflective writing to teach empathy. Academic Medicine. 2004;79(4):351-6.
12. Kleinman A. The illness narratives: Suffering, healing, and the human condition. Basic books; 1988.
13. Charon R. What to do with stories The sciences of narrative medicine. Canadian Family Physician. 2007;53(8):1265-7.
14. Bleakley A. Stories as data, data as stories: making sense of narrative inquiry in clinical education. Medical education. 2005;39(5):534-40.
15. Brown R, Griggs M, Cummins J, Nittler J, Gordy-Panhorst K, Hoffman KG. What Can a Brief Narrative Exercise Reveal About Medical Students' Development as Patient-Centered Physicians and Their Attitudes Toward Patients with Mental Illness? Academic Psychiatry. 2015;39(3):324-8.
16. Deen SR, Mangurian C, Cabaniss DL. Points of contact: Using first-person narratives to help foster empathy in psychiatric residents. Academic Psychiatry. 2010;34(6):438-41.
17. Aronson L, Niehaus B, DeVries CD, Siegel JR, O'Sullivan PS. Do writing and storytelling skill influence assessment of reflective ability in medical students' written reflections? Academic Medicine. 2010;85(10):S29-S32.
18. Law S. Using narratives to trigger reflection. Clin Teach. 2011;8(3):147-50.
19. Brennan N, Corrigan O, Allard J, Archer J, Barnes R, Bleakley A, et al. The transition from medical student to junior doctor: today's experiences of Tomorrow's Doctors. Medical education. 2010;44(5):449-58.
20. Jankouskas TS, Haidet KK, Hupcey JE, Kolanowski A, Murray WB. Targeted crisis resource management training improves performance among randomized nursing and medical students. Simul. 2011;6(6):316-26.

21. Weng HC, Hung CM, Liu YT, Cheng YJ, Yen CY, Chang CC, et al. Associations between emotional intelligence and doctor burnout, job satisfaction and patient satisfaction. Medical education. 2011;45(8):835-42.

22. Keijsers GJ, Schaufeli WB, Le Blanc PM, Zwerts C, Miranda DR. Performance and burnout in intensive care units. Work & Stress. 1995;9(4):513-27.

23. Wallace JE, Lemaire JB, Ghali WA. Physician wellness: a missing quality indicator. Lancet. 2009;374(9702):1714-21.

24. Shanafelt TD, Sloan JA, Habermann TM. The well- being of physicians. The American journal of medicine. 2003;114(6):513-9.

25. Baruch JM. Doctors as Makers. Acad Med. 2017;92(1):40-4.

26. Thompson T, Lamont-Robinson C, Younie L. 'Compulsory creativity': rationales, recipes, and results in the placement of mandatory creative endeavour in a medical undergraduate curriculum. Med. 2010;15.

27. Jowsey T. Musings from an academic kiwi. Auckland: Compassion Publishers; 2016.

28. Compact Oxford English dictionary. Compact Oxford English Dictionary, Oxford: Oxford University Press; 2017 [updated 2017; cited 2013 17.01.2013]. Available from: https://en.oxforddictionaries.com/definition/metaphor

29. Bullough G. Narrative and Dramatic Sources of Shakespeare: Major tragedies. Hamlet, Othello, King Lear, Macbeth. Volume VII. Vol. 7. Columbia University Press; 1973.

30. Steen GJ. From linguistic form to conceptual structure in five steps: analyzing metaphor in poetry. Cognitive poetics. 2009:197-226.

31. Weller J, Boyd M, Cumin D. Teams, tribes and patient safety: overcoming barriers to effective teamwork in healthcare. Postgraduate medical journal. 2014 Mar 1;90(1061):149-54.

32. Best, E. Forest Lore of the Maori. Wellington: Government Printer. 1977.

33. Pihama L, Cram F, Walker S. Creating methodological space: A literature review of Kaupapa Maori research. Canadian Journal of Native Education. 2002 Jan 1;26(1):30.

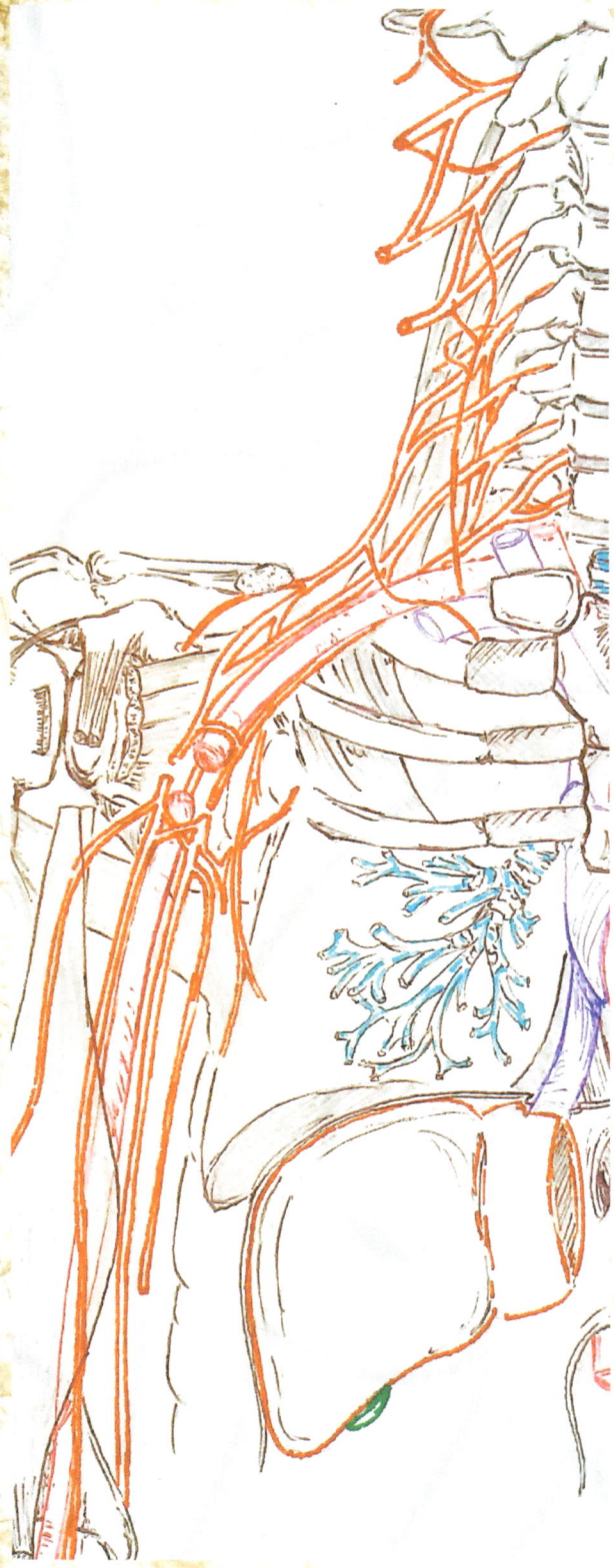

"This book makes clear that our future doctors have heart. It speaks through the beat of poetry and the beauty of art."

Prof. Helen Sword, *author of Stylish Academic Writing*

The importance of the arts in medicine is being increasingly acknowledged in medical programmes the world over. This collection of art and poetry from medical students at the University of Auckland in Aotearoa, New Zealand celebrates their experiences of learning about medicine in practice. Their works are hard-hitting, empathetic, measured, and heart-warming. As a collection, they contribute to a growing global literary discourse of narrative medicine and critical reflection. Journey into their medicine reflections.

Edited by Dr. Tanisha Jowsey, The University of Auckland.

ISBN 978-0-9874920-5-0

9 780987 492050

www.ingramcontent.com/pod-product-compliance
Lightning Source LLC
Chambersburg PA
CBHW041443210326
41599CB00004B/110